Health: The foundations for achievement

David Seedhouse
University of Auckland, New Zealand
and
University of Liverpool, UK

JOHN WILEY & SONS
Chichester · New York · Brisbane · Toronto · Singapore

Library of Congress Cataloging in Publication Data:

Seedhouse, David.
   Health: the foundations for achievement.
   Includes index.
   1. Health. I. Title. II. Series. (DNLM: 1. Health.
QT 255 S451h)
RA776.S445   1986   613   86-5477

ISBN 0 471 91035 X (pbk.)

British Library Cataloguing in Publication Data:

Seedhouse, David
   Health: the foundations for achievement.
   1. Health
   I. Title
   613   RA776
ISBN 0 471 91035 X

Printed and Bound in Great Britain by
Dotesios Ltd, Trowbridge, Wiltshire

Health: The foundations for achievement

*This book is dedicated to the memory of Mum and Dad,
and Ted Dawson—my mentor. It was written for Marilyn,
for whom I wish the best of health always*

There are also Idols formed by the intercourse and association of men with each other, which I call Idols of the Market-place, on account of the commerce and consort of men there. For it is by discourse that men associate; and words are imposed according to the apprehension of the vulgar. And therefore the ill and unfit choice of words wonderfully obstructs the understanding. Nor do the definitions or explanations wherewith in some things learned men are wont to guard and defend themselves, by any means set the matter right. But words plainly force and overrule the understanding, and throw all into confusion, and lead men away into numberless empty controversies and idle fancies.

—Francis Bacon

What then is time? If no-one asks me I know: if I wish to explain it to one that asks, I know not . . . .

—St Augustine

Contents

Contents

Preface

This book poses two fundamental questions. These are: 'What is Health?' and 'How can more health be achieved?' There have been several previous attempts to answer these questions. They form part of a continuing debate which has confusion and ambiguity as its main characteristic. This book, by viewing the debate from a novel perspective, clears away misunderstanding, clarifies the basic issues, and probes the surprising consequences of this clarification.

The book is a gauntlet thrown at the feet of people who claim to be working for health. Although in practice much excellent caring work is done despite this confusion, many 'health workers' have set their sights too low. Disease and illness pose real obstacles to be overcome, but preventing and curing disease and illness is not the whole story of work for health. By working to change only such factors as poor diet and smoking habits, or by prescribing drugs intended to alleviate symptoms brought about by the wider pressures of life, 'health workers' are digging only shallow foundations.

What has emerged from the volumes of writing on health is an indigestible spaghetti of confusion. The word 'health' is already defined in dictionaries, and used everyday as if it is fully understood. In Britain there is a National Health Service and a Minister of Health, there are Health Centres, Health Farms, and academic departments of Health Studies. Health Visitors practise in the community and there are expanding groups working for Health Education and Health Promotion, staffed by professionally qualified Health Education and Health Promotion Officers who devote their careers to increasing health. Consequently it might seem a little late to be asking 'What is Health?' Surely it must be true that people who are working for health know, by definition, what health is.

In spite of all this the fact remains that it is not clear what is being talked about when health is discussed. The word 'health' is used to mean many different things. For a medic health might mean physical fitness, absence of disease, or the harmonious functioning of the organs of the body. For an administrator in a hospital health might mean the state of a person when that person is discharged; for a member of the World Health Organization health might mean complete physical, social and mental wellbeing; for a health educator health might be essentially a freedom to make choices about personal habits and activities, and for a social scientist health might mean a person's ability to function according to social customs and norms — or it might mean the opposite of this if the scientist does not think these norms desirable. Much depends upon the particular profession or interest of whoever is seeking health. Different professions work with different theories of health, and in turn these theories may not be the same as those of the lay people they are trying to serve.

Does a person's health depend on where he lives? Does a person's health depend upon the sort of society in which she lives? Does health vary according to a person's gender? Or according to a person's race? Or according to a person's age? Do doctors work for full health? Is the National Health Service a misnomer? It is possible to study for a Diploma of Health Education at some British Polytechnics, but even on these courses it is not made fully clear what health education actually is, or should be.

These and many other questions need to be tackled urgently, and the web of confusion that has been fostered by ambiguity must be untangled. The extent of the ambiguity can be disconcerting. People expect to be able to specify the nature of health. If the symptoms of illnesses and diseases can be described fairly precisely it is natural to think that health too ought to be describable in a fairly precise way. However, it is not so easy; issues about the nature of health are complicated and contentious. 'Health' is one of a number of words which are constantly in use which are so rich in meaning that they cannot be explained fully without invoking controversy. This poses a challenge for us to try to understand more clearly what we mean when we use such words, and to pinpoint limits beyond which we do not wish to use them. To understand the problems involved and to arrive at a proper view of the full sense of health requires effort. It is not possible, even if it were desirable, to lead a student of health by the hand to an indisputable conclusion. The student must work to see the point of alternative theories, to recognize the difficulties involved with each, and then to arrive at a considered opinion.

The primary aim of this book is to clarify the meanings and sense of the word 'health'. It is naturally appealing to try to change the human condition by a frontal attack, to try to cure injustice, poverty, sickness, drabness, and the inhuman treatment of people by their fellow men with urgent action, but the track record of previous such interventions is not good. Cautious preparation is essential. It is far better first to clarify the ground from which to work, to know that what is to be said has been thoroughly thought through, and that the position can be properly defended against attack. This is the reason for doing philosophy. This is a central aim of this book.

Because of this need for a careful preparation some patience is required to read the book. At times the discussion is almost purely theoretical. Such puzzling about abstract issues may irritate practitioners who are used to trying to solve urgent problems by direct action. Even though the approach of the book is at all times appropriate to real problems of life one objection will inevitably be raised. This is one version of it:

> 'We know what is wrong with society and the British health service already. Why bother with the preliminaries? Why write this sort of book at all?
>
> 'What is the point of writing a book that tries first and foremost to get to the roots of meaning and sense of a single word? Surely there are many more relevant directions along which to press an inquiry than to pursue abstract clarification and discussion of ideas. Our world is beset by real problems which are clear enough already. Within and between societies there are gross inequalities of wealth, power, quality of life, opportunity, food and housing resources. Enormous sums of money are spent on military research and on arming some nations with a thousand-times more destructive power than is needed to annihilate the entire Earth, while at the same time people are dying of starvation. Only a privileged few are able to develop themselves intellectually by attending centres of higher education, while others go through life only barely literate

and numerate, either to work long hours for low pay—or not to work at all; and our world is suffering from the pollution of land, sea, and air as a result of short-sighted industrial policies and processes.'

There are so many blatant wrongs to be righted that scepticism about the worth of an investigation into a word—six black letters on a white page—seems fully justified. Such scepticism might be appropriate if the pursuit of health was abandoned following clarification, but the clarifying process is only one part of the project. Because of the work done to clear the ground properly it becomes possible to put forward a more precise and comprehensive theory of health than has ever been offered before.

Health should be thought of as *the foundations for achievement*. Health is not a single goal which can be universally achieved—health has degrees and levels just as different sorts of buildings have different sorts and standards of foundations. These foundations are not merely those required for biological or physical achievement. They are those required for a wide range of human achievement, including the biological but also encompassing emotional, intellectual, spiritual, creative, and recreational potentials. Some of the foundations which make up a person's health are essential to enable any human being to achieve anything worthwhile.

The implications of this new theory of health are huge. To win the battle for fuller health there must be major changes in the education system, in freedom of access to information, and in the system of basic welfare in societies. Health is already a significant political issue, but the issue is far more explosive than many who advocate the dismantling or the expansion of the health service, or existing systems of 'health care' in other societies, realize.

Acknowledgements

I would like to thank my friends, Alan Cribb and Harry Lesser, all the members of the Oldham WEA philosophy group who endured my ramblings and misconceptions about health, Dr Michael Wilson and Dr Rosemary Biggs. All challenged my ideas and pointed out better directions to take.

Chapter One
What is Health?

The Challenge

The challenge is clear. The task is to discover what health means and then to explain how more of it can be achieved. The first target is to answer the question 'What is Health?'

There are a variety of uses of the word, and a number of possible definitions. A person can say that he 'has health' now, or that he 'is healthy' in general. He can say that he has 'mental health' or 'functional health'. He can claim to have a 'healthy appetite', a 'healthy attitude towards life', and that he lives in a 'healthy society'. A person can be a 'health educator', eat 'health food' and work in a department of 'health studies'. She can insist that she is healthy because she lives in a democracy, or a family, or a community. Or that she possesses 'spiritual health' because she is a Christian.

It is possible to argue that the correct definition of health is either that *health is a commodity* to be given and possessed, or that *health is a particular ideal state*, or that *health is a variable state which enables a person to function normally*, or that *health is a reserve of strength*, or that *health is an ability to adapt to changing circumstances*, or that *health is a resilient spirit*. The present task is to discover a way out of this maze. Which of these uses and definitions are important, and which are trivial? Is there a thread which links them all? What is common to them?

Two points must be made clear from the outset. These are as follows.

1. To discover the meaning of health it is not enough to consult a dictionary

The issue is not as simple as this. Dictionaries are not oracles. The people who compile dictionaries are not in a privileged position of absolute authority where the meanings of words are concerned. Dictionaries are written by people from particular societies and eras who have particular sets and sorts of values and beliefs. It is perfectly possible to disagree with dictionary definitions and to provide good reasons for doing so. This is illustrated by the fact that there are so many different theories and ideas about health. The writer Raymond Williams has demonstrated this point very well. He said that:

> Some people, when they see a word, think the first thing to do is define it. Dictionaries are produced and, with a show of authority no less confident because it is so limited in place and time, what is called a proper meaning is attached. I once began collecting,

from correspondence in newspapers, and from other public arguments, variations on the phrases 'I see from my Webster' and 'I find from my Oxford dictionary'. Usually what was at issue was a difficult term in an argument. But the effective tone of these phrases, with their interesting overture of possession ('my Webster'), was to appropriate a meaning which fitted the argument and to exclude those meanings which were inconvenient to it but which some benighted person had been so foolish as to use. Of course if we want to be clear about . . . *barber*, or *barley*, or *barn*, this kind of definition is effective. But for words of a different kind, and especially for those which involve ideas and values, it is not only an impossible but an irrelevant procedure. (Williams, 1976, pp. 14-15)

The idea of health is not to be found within the pages of any dictionary. The idea of health is disputed. Not all people are of the same opinion about health. Different views can be held legitimately.

The history of the word 'health' is that it was first used to indicate 'wholeness'. To this extent a study of dictionaries is useful because an initial limit is fixed. The limit is very vague however. What does the idea of 'wholeness' mean in practice? What does a person who is not whole look like? What is a whole person? Dictionaries set a very basic stage on which to work. They do not answer important questions, they help to form them.

2. It is not enough to say that health is desirable, and to leave the issue there

The following inadequate position can be advanced. It is common knowledge that people have different values—after all, this is what politics is all about—and that these values depend on such factors as their education, friends, experiences, families, and societies. This means that people are bound to have different goals and will prefer to spend their time in different ways. *In order to do these things people need their health.* Health is essential to people's fulfilment. Since this is the case all that has to be said is that *health is desirable.* This is the end of the matter. Health does mean different things to different people but *nobody wants bad health.*

Such a position has recently been adopted by a British university. In a course entitled *Health and Disease* (Open University, 1985) there is a small section on 'The Concept of Health' which briefly, and arbitrarily, discusses several alternative 'concepts', 'notions' and 'definitions'. The author of the section, who is unnamed, concludes that '. . . the terms "health" and "healthy" can be applied to every aspect of human life, depending on the values of the speaker; indeed they may function simply as a way of praising anything one happens to like.' In a very weak sense this is true, but this is a thoroughly unsatisfactory position to put forward in a whole year's course to be spent studying health issues. Would we be justified in calling such diverse things as the murder of Jews in gas ovens, rape, weapons research, Socialism, Toryism, smoking, and butter 'healthy' if we like these things and want to praise them? Students of the course cannot be sure what the values of the course authors are, and so will not know what they are talking about when they mention 'health'.

Such lazy thinking leads the inquiry nowhere. Although it is not wrong to say that health is desirable the phrase conveys very little of substance about the nature of health. The problem is that what one person actively desires, another person may actively be trying to avoid.

It does not help us form a satisfactory understanding of what health is to say that it is desirable. Once the phrase 'that which is desirable' is used in practice rather than cast in abstract terms it becomes apparent that *actual goals (personal desires) need not be desired universally*. Not all human beings have the same hierarchy of desires. In any case where desires seem to be 'obviously universal' there will always be people who have good reasons not to desire what the majority desire.

For example, on the face of it it seems obvious that all human beings will desire to be free from disease and illness. The following three points show that this is not obvious:

1. Some diseases can be culturally defined so that what is regarded as a disease in one culture will be regarded as normal and desirable in another. Lester King has given the example of foot-binding in China, when women suffered pain and disability in order to be fashionable, but were not considered to be diseased or ill in any way. In British society these women would be considered to be injured at least.
2. It is well known that there are cases in which disease and illness is desired and even encouraged in order to avoid work, or to engender sympathy, or to obtain privilege.
3. People can be prepared to accept disease and illness in order to achieve what they consider to be higher goals, while other people with different values can wish to be free of disease and illness at all costs. An example of the former type is an individual who is a famine relief worker who expects to contract some sort of tropical disease or illness as a part of his work. This person actually desires a state—being a relief worker in a foreign country—which will inevitably lead to a state which the latter individual is determined to avoid.

The discussion has already become too abstract. Can the question 'What is Health?' best be answered at the level of everyday life?

When is a Person Healthy?

Health is indisputably to do with people. The best approach must be to look at people in everyday circumstances, to examine real lives. If it is then possible to say that some people are healthy and other people are not this must provide good clues about what health means. The grounds for the decision that a person is either healthy or not will be assessable, and from this analysis it should be possible to construct a clear general theory of health.

The case studies

None of these studies is of an actual person, but each is drawn from the experiences of real people. The studies are presented to provoke thought. They are designed to confront those who think they know what health is but cannot really be bothered to put it into words because it is so obvious. After each study the following questions should be asked.

Is the person healthy? If he is, why is he? If he is not, why is he unhealthy?

Percy Percy is a thirty-six year old white bachelor. In the past he has worked as a clerk in three offices. He was responsible for the sale and despatch of spare parts for cranes. Six years ago he was made redundant by his company because of the prevailing economic recession, and because his work could be done more efficiently by the firm's computer. Since then he has had to make do with various kinds of temporary work, usually manual, and he has had to draw unemployment benefit if nothing else was available. Three years ago Percy began to suffer from occasional delusions over which he had no control. He would believe that he was another person. He would take on that person's character, and act exactly as if he were that person and had that person's role. Sometimes the people he imagined himself to be were real and known to him. At other times they were invented. The delusions never lasted longer than three hours, and afterwards Percy could remember nothing about what had happened.

Once Percy acted as if he was the office manager at the company he had worked for as a twenty year old. One lunchtime he took over a desk at the office of the builder by whom he was employed as a temporary labourer and managed to order eight jib sections of cranes which were then invoiced to the building firm. On another occasion he believed he was Bruce Springsteen—a hero of long-standing—and ran up an overdraft by spending £1500 at various clothing and musical instrument shops.

Recently Percy has sought professional help. He knows that he cannot expect to hold down a job if his present problem continues, since his sporadic delusions make it impossible for people to treat him as a normal person. At the time of each delusion no-one can communicate with Percy. They have to interact with Bruce, or whoever else he is at the time. Percy consulted his GP who referred him to a psychiatrist. Both doctors could find nothing physically wrong with Percy. He has no disease which medical science can label with certainty. It has been suggested to Percy that he become a voluntary patient at the local hospital for mental illness.

Dennis Dennis is a forty-five year old white man. He has worked as a bank clerk for twenty years, and he has worked at his present branch for eight years. He is rather flabby but he is not overweight according to the norm for his height and body structure. He is married and lives in a smallish three-bedroomed semi-detached house on an estate built just before the Second World War. He has no children.

Dennis returns home from work each day and can do no more than eat his evening meal—which is always prepared for him by his wife—and then doze in front of the television before retiring to bed. At weekends Dennis likes to 'lie-in' until at least midday. He enjoys watching the sports programmes that are on television on Saturday and Sunday afternoons. Dennis visits his local GP once a year for a check-up. He has no diseases and does not feel ill.

Anne Anne is a white woman of thirty-two. She had been working as a journalist for a women's magazine before suffering a serious car accident. A vehicle overtaking from the opposite direction forced her off the road, making her collide at speed with a solid brick wall. She had enjoyed her work, which involved writing special features and travelling to report from the scene of news events. She is now a paraplegic—her lower limbs and part of her torso are paralysed. She lives in a specially designed flat, on her own since her husband left her saying that she is not the woman she was. And yet she is now content, caring, and always tries to encourage others, whatever their problem. She receives help from health and social service workers, provided by the State from tax revenue.

She has a good income from the interest from the compensation she received from the insurers of the driver of the car that caused her to crash, and from payment for various articles which she writes regularly for various magazines on a freelance basis. She now specializes in writing for periodicals for the disabled, and in writing for feminist publications about social policy.

Betty Betty is white, and a widow of fifty-one. She has three children, two of whom are married and have left home. She lives in a house, which she owns outright, with her youngest son who is sixteen. He is taking 'A' Levels at the local technical college.

Betty has cancer. Two years ago she had a mastectomy which was followed by a course of radiation therapy, and then by chemotherapy. She has been feeling ill recently and has been told that cancer has reappeared as a small but inoperable tumour on her brain. Once again she is having radiation therapy, which is again to be followed by a course of chemotherapy. On top of her headaches and increasing immobility she knows that she will feel intermittent nausea and that her new crop of hair will all fall out as a result of her treatment.

Betty is miserable and very frightened, as much about what will become of her young son, who is now stealing, lying, and not doing any academic work, than about what will happen to her. However, despite all this she is showing great character and has resolved to fight her disease with all the strength she has. She is determined to survive, at least until she has seen her son move successfully into adult life — something which she knows may take several years.

The James family Mr and Mrs James are both white and aged twenty. They are living in a thirteenth-floor council flat which has walls which are peeling because of damp in one bedroom. Their electricity supply has recently been cut off because of non-payment of substantial arrears. Mrs James had an abortion nine months ago. Six weeks ago she took an overdose of Valium, and last week was found by her GP to be pregnant. When she was a very small child she spent nine weeks 'in care', after which she was brought up by her step-mother. She feels very depressed and frequently says that she cannot go on any more and that life is bound to get even worse for her.

Mr James is currently on probation for car theft and for house-breaking. He has never had paid employment in his life and, although he has tried, he has been unable to get a job. Their only child is three-and-a-half years old. His speech is slow and he has recurrent bronchitis. He also has frequent temper tantrums.

Winston Winston is twenty-two, black — of West Indian stock — and British. He has lived in a small, damp, terraced house in Moss Side, Manchester, all his life. In the summer of 1989 he, like all his friends, was involved in riots in Moss Side and Rusholme. The reason for the riots was that black kids were protesting against their lack of opportunity, and against the way they felt they were being treated unfairly by the predominantly white local police force. Winston was arrested and charged with obstructing the police. He claimed that he had merely been watching the disturbances and the fires. He was found guilty. Since then he is regularly taken into Moss Side police station for questioning about his activities. In common with most of his friends Winston has never had a full-time job. He deals in 'soft drugs' in a small way in order to supplement his benefit. So far this has been overlooked by the police although Winston is sure they know what he is doing. Winston has a fine physique. He is in excellent physical shape because he works out everyday at the local sports centre.

Peter   Peter is a fifty-three year old white man. He is married with two daughters, both of whom are studying at university. He is a successful businessman who owns his own company trading in cut-glass for the upper range of the market. He lives in a luxurious detached house, standing in an acre of grounds which are looked after by a gardener whom Peter employs for two days per week. He has a good circle of friends and acquaintances, he enjoys golf, and he is active in the local branch of the Conservative Party. He lives the 'good life' to the full. He smokes thirty good quality cigarettes a day, often supplemented with two or three cigars. He eats most things heartily but does try to keep his weight down since he cares about his appearance. He drinks two or three pints of beer—always 'real ale'—per day, as well as three or four whisky 'chasers'.
He is still very ambitious and becomes frustrated easily. Occasionally this frustration becomes manifest in a fit of temper, and twice in the past year he has struck his wife in the face with the palm of his hand.

Which of these people are healthy and which are unhealthy?

In order to reach conclusions about the state of health of these people we need to have some idea about what health is, but no clear idea of health springs from the descriptions of these people's lives.

   There are two options open. One is to try different existing definitions of health to see how they work out. The other is to attempt a personal assessment of the case studies in order to say that person X seems to be healthier than person Y, and then to work out why. Neither of these alternatives can provide a clear-cut answer to the question 'What is Health?'

1.   To take the first option, consider the answers which might be given by four hypothetical people who each hold a different definition of health. These people are a medic, a social scientist, an idealist from the World Health Organization, and a Humanist. This particular medic defines health as *the absence of disease, illness and injury*. The social scientist defines health as *the ability to function in a normal social role*. The idealist defines health as *a state of complete physical, mental and social well-being*. And this particular humanist thinks that health is *an ability to adapt positively to the problems of life*.

The medic   According to the medic *Percy is unhealthy* because he is ill. Although she cannot put a name to Percy's illness she thinks it highly likely that someone will be able to. In any case, Percy certainly is not normal. *Dennis is healthy*, although he does seem to be excessively idle. *Anne is unhealthy*—it makes no sense to describe a cripple as healthy. *Betty is unhealthy* because she has cancer. *Mrs James is probably unhealthy* since she is so depressed. *Mr James is healthy. The James child is unhealthy. Winston is very healthy*—he is very fit. *Peter is healthy*, although he should watch his smoking and drinking.

The social scientist The problem for the social scientist is to define what a normal social role is. According to this scientist it is what a person has been functioning as for the last three years in which they had no serious disease, illness or injury unusual to them. The social scientist thinks that *Percy is unhealthy* because he is not functioning in his normal social role. *Dennis is healthy. Anne has regained her health. Betty is unhealthy* because she is unable to do what she used to. *The James family are healthy*—they have had their social roles for over three years. *Winston is healthy* because he has an established way of life. *Peter is healthy* because he has an important social role.

The idealist As far as the idealist is concerned *they are all unhealthy.*

The humanist The humanist has his own ideas about what positive adaptation is. He thinks that most people will agree with him. In his opinion *Percy is healthy* since he is doing what he can to cure himself of his delusions. *Dennis is unhealthy* because he is drifting and doing nothing positive to change his unfulfilling life. *Anne is healthy* because she has adapted excellently to her considerable disabilities. *Betty is healthy* because she is responding positively to her disease and her circumstances. *The James family is unhealthy. Winston is healthy* because he is doing all the positive things he knows. Although in the opinion of this humanist he could be a lot healthier if he channelled his energies in other directions. He thinks *Peter is unhealthy* because he does not consider wife-beating to be a positive adaptation to stress.

All this is messy and perplexing. Percy, Betty, Mrs James and the James child have been described as unhealthy three times, and as healthy once. Dennis, Anne, Mr James and Peter have each been labelled healthy twice and unhealthy twice. Winston has been described as healthy three times and as unhealthy once.

The discussion of these case studies clearly highlights the problem that health means different things to different people.

2. The second option is to attempt a personal assessment of the lives described, without having a definition beforehand. Many people have tried this. The most common outcome is puzzlement.

People are usually dissatisfied with the answers given by those who have definite set ideas about health. What is wrong is that the issues are falsely cast in black and white. Health issues do not seem to boil down to questions of either/or. Most people want to conclude that most of the case studies are *healthy in some respects* even though they are unhealthy in others. For example, Anne does not seem to have physical health but she has excellent mental and emotional health. Winston has marvellous physical health but seems badly unfulfilled intellectually and emotionally. Betty is not healthy physically because she has secondary cancer, but she is showing so much resolve, mental strength, stamina, and courage that she surely has a high standard of mental wellbeing.

This way of looking at the case studies seems to be a more balanced and flexible approach, but it has not advanced the inquiry far because it allows the statement that *a person can be healthy and unhealthy at the same time*. As things stand this appears to be a clear contradiction, on a par with the statement that a person can both be diseased and not diseased at the same time. Later it will become clear that this is not the case, but the problem now is that we are attempting to answer the question 'What is Health?' at a stage which is too early in the investigation. We are not properly prepared, and we do not have a specific theory to test. In order to get to the bottom of the issue, in order to defeat the frustration felt at not being able to answer a question which is superficially very simple, it is first necessary to step back from it. It is necessary to see the importance of clarification, to appreciate the extent of the problem of meaning, and to recognize the merits and problems of existing theories of health.

Chapter Two
The Need for Philosophy

Although departments of philosophy in British universities are currently being run down, and even closed altogether, there remains and will always remain a real need for philosophy in our intellectual and practical lives. Some people see no need for a discipline which takes the time to reflect on what is happening around it, which tries to focus issues sharply, and then to suggest what could be done to change things for the better. Some people would rather, arrogantly, continue to do what they have always done because *they know* that they are right. However, it is always better to take the time to examine alternatives, and to be willing to change course if necessary. Nobody can be right all the time.

We have been trying to answer the question 'What is Health?', and we have run into difficulties. It is as if we have stepped from what we thought was solid rock into a shifting quicksand. There are so many competing opinions and ideas about health that it seems almost impossible to decide which are good and which are poor, which are useful and which are red herrings. It is in situations such as this that philosophical activity is necesssary.

Philosophers are sometimes criticized for thinking in a vacuum. They are accused of abstracting ideas out of the practical world, and then playing trivial intellectual games with them. The charge is occasionally made against philosophy that there is no point in trying to work things out *aculturally* and *ahistorically*. Without the context of the real world the ideas that are toyed with are meaningless.

Sometimes such criticisms are justified, but they are not always correct, and the polar opposite approach can be criticized in turn. Never to take ideas out of the stream of practical life is short-sighted and leads only to blinkered single-mindedness. All the thinking done by people who are convinced by certain theories which refer only to historical and cultural contexts can serve only to reinforce their existing convictions about the theories they believe in. This happens frequently with political dogma and dogmatists.

In fact, many people do philosophy without realizing it. When people change their opinions, when they begin to see the strength of views which they previously thought to be worthless, when blurred ideas become sharper, then people are doing philosophy.

How can philosophy help in the inquiry into the nature of health? A full answer to the question 'What is Health?' can be given only by standing back from the various disputes to take the widest possible view. This degree of detachment can be achieved only with great difficulty, if at all, by the disciplines which already favour one particular meaning or set of meanings of health over other possibilities. The problem is that the practitioners within relevant disciplines have beliefs which inevitably predispose them to particular views about health. It is not that a social scientist will see only social factors affecting health, or that a biologist will see only biological factors. The point is more subtle than this. A specialist will be inclined by her experience and training to look for certain factors which she will regard as more pertinent than others, and she will be equipped to describe and explain a situation in a particular way. She will have to make decisions about which information is most worthy of inclusion and this judgement will be influenced by her background (see appendix for an expansion of this point).

This investigation into the meaning of health has uncovered a tricky problem. There seems to be a paradox that *health is a goal which is desired universally, but which does not have a universally shared meaning, and so cannot be desired universally.* Philosophy can solve this paradox because its concern is elucidation. Philosophy aims to be as detached as it is possible to be in any inquiry, in order to have the clearest view of the issues.

This lack of direct involvement that is needed to do philosophy can be seen as a weakness. What does health have to do with philosophy? It is often taken for granted that health is the concern of practical people, and of no interest to philosophers. It is generally assumed that health is something which is promoted, encouraged, prescribed for, or studied. It is achieved by exercise, moderation, good diet, drugs, and surgery. Health is the exclusive concern of the professionals who work at the sharp end of research and practice. Health is the goal of medics, biologists, psychologists, chemists, statisticians, nurses, health visitors, and health educators. It is a legitimate area of study for historians, sociologists, political scientists, economists, and geographers, but it is not the concern of philosophy.

It is argued that philosophers are experts at debating metaphysical issues (for instance, about different ways of classifying what can be known), experts at resolving questions about what counts as legitimate knowledge (for instance, deciding between what is known and what is merely believed), and experts at assessing which methods of inquiry are sound, and what arrangements of propositions are valid (one aspect of logic). It is sometimes felt that the nearest philosophers can get to practical problems is in their discussions of moral issues, and that even then they are mainly interested in the production or discovering of basic moral rules (meta-ethics), so leaving the solution of particular ethical dilemmas to those who are most directly affected—in medicine there are 'ethical committees' who do not use philosophers. The prevailing opinion is that philosophy should stick to its proper place and allow other specialisms to do the same.

Not everyone takes this view. There are exceptions, but versions of this opinion are relatively common. Those who hold it do not understand what true philosophy is.

What is Philosophy?

As in all other things, this view of philosophy will not be shared by everyone.

Philosophy is clarification

The philosopher Ludwig Wittgenstein wrote:

Philosophy aims at the logical clarification of thoughts.
Philosophy is not a body of doctrine but an activity.
A philosophical work consists essentially of elucidations.
Philosophy does not result in 'philosophical propositions', but rather in the clarification of propositions.
Without philosophy thoughts are, as it were, cloudy and indistinct: its task is to make them clear and to give them sharp boundaries. (Wittgenstein, 1974, p. 112)

Wittgenstein's point is that philosophy aims to clear away confusion through tight analysis. But it is not necessarily true that all thoughts should be given sharp boundaries if they do not actually have such boundaries. Some thoughts are naturally fuzzy.

Philosophy is not a production line creating ideas which always lead to practical solutions to definite problems. Philosophy can help the achievement of practical solutions to problems, but the activity will not necessarily have this effect. Philosophy is not a mechanism by which dogmatism is created, nor is it a board on which ideologies can be pinned. True philosophy is not 'being philosophical' in the sense of resigning oneself to one's fate—it is the opposite of this. True philosophy does not involve having a general policy—where there are certain acknowledged dos and don'ts—such as is described by the 'philosophy of management'. Nor is true philosophy the same as 'having a philosophy' in the sense of having a specific set of ideas. Philosophical activity is more concerned with retaining the awareness that clarifications are incomplete than it is with obtaining 'the right answers'.

Philosophy is essentially the act of attempting clarification. It is a personal activity. The tangible end-product of a particular philosophical labour can often seem trite. It might result in a statement which was known already. It may be something which has taken thousands of words to explain but which apparently can be said as well in a single sentence. It may even be that this end-product could be arrived at by a less painful method. But if so then it will not be the same end-product, even though in isolation from the philosopher it is identical in every respect. Philosophy demands much from the philosopher. It demands an intense personal involvement with fundamental questions which cannot be let go and which must be pressed as far as possible. Philosophy involves asking questions which are perhaps thought by some people to be too obvious to ask. Philosophy is concerned with asking such questions repeatedly and rigorously. It is a personal fight for clarity. Philosophy is a personal struggle—a wrestling match in which you are never certain that you have an opponent other than yourself. Philosophy is a process of self-education. Philosophy cannot be taught in the way that language, science or geography can, but because it clarifies it can inspire philosophy in others. Philosophy is a process which develops a person. It is not something which can be passed on second-hand, although *the results* of the activity can.

Children are philosophers

We all have philosophical ability, but for pragmatic reasons, because it is generally felt that in order to function any society requires answers, certainty, and assurance, philosophy is inexorably kicked out of us. The questions of some children are condemned as 'childish questions' although they are the questions of philosophers.

'What does God look like?', 'Why must I go to school?', 'Am I healthy?', 'Why does rain come in drops?', 'Why must I die?' . . . 'Why?' . . . 'Why?' At first, people cannot help but try to dispel clouds with their curiosity. Before people learn to think of it as a jokey game, before they have grown to expect evasions and conventional answers, they are never satisfied. These sorts of question are honest. They stem from a genuine puzzlement, and we should never stop asking them.

An example from Plato

Plato knew this, as this illustration from *The Republic* shows.

The main thread which runs through *The Republic* is the search for the meaning of 'justice'. On the face of it the meaning of 'justice' seems clear enough, but on analysis the issue is shown to be very complicated. Several definitions of justice are suggested. Socrates squeezes out the sense and implications of each suggestion in order to test them for adequacy. At one point the question 'what is justice?' is cast in the form 'who is a just man?' It is suggested that a just man is one who tells the truth and pays his debts. But is this so in all cases? Socrates asks, should one return arms to a madman?

Polemachus, his intellectual adversary at the time, responds, 'No, not in that case, not if the parties are friends and evil would result. He [Simonides—the original proposer of the idea] meant that you were to do what was proper, good to friends and harm to enemies.' But the view that justice does good to friends and harm to enemies will not do for Socrates for several reasons. Among these is the point that it is not necessarily the case that our friends are good and our enemies evil, and the further point that it is likely that if evil is rendered to the evil this will serve only to make the evil more evil still.

This process of debate continues throughout *The Republic*. No final satisfactory definition is reached—and this is an important lesson.

Anyone can do philosophy without needing qualifications or having taken any courses in the subject. So what is unique about philosophy? It is the realization that there are no questions which cannot or should not be asked, and that there is no end to questioning. To do philosophy personal intellectual insecurity is a great strength if it is coupled with a stubborn energy and patience. Where other approaches reach answers with which they can be satisfied, at least temporarily, philosophy continues to force questions because of a personal compulsion. This does not mean that a philosopher cannot produce a theory. Philosophy is not an affliction, nor is it a process which leaves no room for any other thought, but it does mean that a philosopher will never believe his theory to be a complete or final answer. He will criticize it and attempt to change and improve it as often as he can.

There are sound reasons why we should all exercise our philosophical abilities, even if this involves shifting a lot of dust.

1. We should all practise clarification. We should cultivate a systematic bloody-mindedness. We owe it to ourselves, if we are thinking, autonomous people, not to take anything at face value until we have thought it through personally.
2. Where our work affects other people, as is the case with work for health, it is vital to recognize that not everyone has the same values and priorities. We must

work to clarify what the priorities of other people are, without imposing our own.

Such questions as these should become habits.

What am I trying to do when I work to help people, and when I promote health? Does this person want what I regard as health? For example, to be relieved of cancer temporarily at the expense of hair loss and nausea is not everyone's idea of a route to health. Neither is stopping smoking at the cost of stress, family rows, and depression. How am I influencing him? How can I tell what she wants? Is he capable of telling me? If not—if he is a young child or senile—how else can I find out?

Chapter Three
The Problem of Meaning

A prospective employer requests the opinion of a qualified physician on the present state of health of Mr Smith, a candidate for a job. Mr Smith is told that a physical examination is not required, but instead is asked some questions by the physician. The doctor asks about Mr Smith's 'general health'. Mr Smith replies that it is 'fine'. The doctor asks about Mr Smith's diet, to which Mr Smith, thinking immediately of fried fish and chips and white bread and butter, assures the doctor that he has a 'healthy appetite'. The doctor inquires whether Mr Smith has 'a healthy social life too, with friends, exercise and conversation?' Mr Smith readily agrees, telling the doctor that he plays football every week. It does not cross his mind to mention that he suffers purgatory at each Sunday morning game as a result of Saturday night's eating and drinking excesses. Finally the doctor asks about Mr Smith's 'emotional state', to which Mr Smith replies that he is 'always happy' and has never been 'mentally ill'. The doctor is satisfied, and so are Mr Smith and his new employer.

This brief tale is sparse, hypothetical and ought to be implausible, but it is not impossible. Beneath its superficiality lie worrying misunderstandings—can a person who is 'always happy' really be 'mentally well'?—and a fundamental question. What, if anything, is communicated in encounters such as this, where words are used with little thought?

Why Should there be Such Difficulty in Pinning Down the Meaning of Health?

We do not fully understand our world, but we naturally assume that we do fully understand the words we have invented to describe and explain it, but this is not so. Because our understanding of the world is imprecise the meanings of many of the words we use are imprecise.

To understand why there should be such difficulty in pinning down the meaning of health it is important to recognize that the problem associated with the word 'health' is not unique. All the important words in the human vocabulary are more vague than is generally realized.

The History of the Word 'Health'

Although it is not sufficient on its own, the history of the meaning of health must be considered.

Health has not always been viewed as a medical speciality. Historically health was associated with 'wholeness'. The etymology of health is that it is derived from the

14

word 'whole'. An etymological dictionary records this brief history, under the general heading 'whole':

> 'OE *hal*, well, has derivative *haelth* (abstract suffix *-th*)—ME *helthe*—E *health*.' (Partridge, 1966, p. 805)

Michael Foucault has written that this notion of 'health' as soundness of body, mind, and spirit prevailed until approximately 200 years ago, at which time the growth of professional medicine began to create changes in thinking about health:

> Generally speaking, it might be said that up to the end of the eighteenth century medicine related much more to health than to normality; it did not begin by analysing a 'regular' functioning of the organism and go on to seek where it had deviated, what it was disturbed by, and how it could be brought back into normal working order; it referred, rather, to qualities of vigour, suppleness and fluidity, which were lost in illness and which it was the task of medicine to restore. To this extent medical practice could accord an important place to regimen and diet, in short to a whole rule of life and nutrition that the subject imposed upon himself. This privileged relation between medicine and health involved the possibility of being one's own physician. Nineteenth century medicine, on the other hand, was regulated more in accordance with normality than with health; it formed its concepts and prescribed its interventions in relation to the standard functioning and organic structure, and physiological knowledge—once marginal and purely theoretical knowledge for the doctor—was to become established . . . at the very centre of all medical reflexion. (Foucault, 1973, p. 35)

Foucault describes a gradual move from regarding health as 'qualities of vigour, suppleness and fluidity' to coming to see it as a state of biological normality which could be achieved by external intervention. Previously health was considered to be an autonomously created 'whole rule of life' rather than something which could be given by another person's intervention, independent of personal effort. There has been a move from health which required personal action to health which can be imposed or acquired—health as a commodity.

The analysis of the history of the word shows the width of meaning that health can have, but it does nothing to dispel the ambiguity. To say that 'to be healthy is to be whole' is not particularly informative. The phrase hides more specific meanings behind an opaque veil created by this fine-sounding word. It also obscures understanding about practical methods of helping more people achieve this wholeness.

Francis Bacon and the Idols of the Market-place

Francis Bacon understood the need for clarity and focus in human thought, and not only where words and meanings are concerned. He knew that human beings construct, either involuntarily or through carelessness, certain barriers against understanding. He described these human defects as being akin to the worship of 'Idols' or false gods. He identified four types: 'Idols of the Tribe', 'Idols of the Cave', 'Idols of the Theatre' and 'Idols of the Market-place'.

When he explained 'The Idols of the Tribe' Bacon was referring to the tendency for all human beings to suppose that their senses give a full and accurate knowledge of reality, and that the order that human beings perceive directly in nature actually exists. Bacon thought that this tendency is a fault. He argued that human perceptions act to distort the information we receive. He described perceptions as 'false mirrors' on reality.

'The Idols of the Cave' are the particular prejudices of each human being, our personal biases which have resulted from our unique experiences, friends, teachers, political views, religious beliefs, and so on. This means that the evidence we receive of external events is always interpreted or adulterated in the light of personally favoured theories. Each of us 'has his own private den or cavern, which intercepts and discolours the light of nature'. Bacon thought that evidence is never pure, but that for it to mean anything to an individual it has to be interpreted, and that this act of interpretation creates what are often wrongly described as 'objective facts' (see Appendix).

The 'Idols of the Theatre' cause the errors which 'have crept into men's minds from the various dogmas and systems of philosophy'. Here Bacon was describing the folly and intellectual stagnation which he believed had been produced by an unthinking adherence to the doctrines of Aristotle, but he was also making the general point that blind acceptance of 'received wisdom' is an empty and destructive obedience.

The most powerful 'Idols' of all are those which still plague us to the highest degree. They are the 'Idols of the Market-place'. They seem to appear in abundance when health issues are discussed. These 'false notions' arise from the exchange and commerce of words. Bacon saw two main dangers naturally associated with the use of words. Firstly many words are ambiguous. Often two people use the same word with a different meaning but fail to realise their mistake. In other words people can talk at 'cross-purposes' and fail to realize this because of misapprehension about what the person with whom they are conversing means by a word. One result of this can be that they think they agree but actually they disagree.

Secondly, words are apt to be taken to represent things. Words which actually stand for nothing concrete are taken to refer to existing entities just because they are written or spoken so frequently. Bacon's examples were 'fortune' and 'prime mover'. 'Mind' might be a further example and so might 'health'.

Many politicians, journalists and students, amongst others, worship these 'Idols' with a regrettable fervour. Solzhenitsyn has explained Bacon's thesis in a powerful way:

> All right, then, let's call it a more refined form of the herd instinct, the fear of remaining alone, *outside the community*. There's nothing new about it. Francis Bacon set out his doctrine of idols back in the sixteenth century. He said that people are not inclined to live by pure experience, that it is easier for them to pollute experience with prejudices. These prejudices are the idols . . .
>
> What are the idols of the theatre?
>
> The idols of the theatre are the authoritative opinions of others which a man likes to accept as a guide when interpreting something he hasn't experienced himself . . . sometimes he actually experienced it, only it's more convenient not to believe what he's seen.
>
> I've seen cases like that as well . . .
>
> Another idol of the theatre is our over-willingness to agree with the arguments of science. One can sum this up as the voluntary acceptance of other people's errors! . . . Finally there are the idols of the market-place.

This was easiest of all to imagine: an alabaster idol towering over a swarming crowd in a market-place.

The idols of the market-place are the errors which result from the communication and association of men with each other. They are the errors a man commits because it has become customary to use certain phrases and formulas which do violence to reason. For example, 'Enemy of the people!' 'Not one of us!' 'Traitor!' Call a man one of these and everyone will renounce him . . .

And over all idols there is the sky of fear, the sky of fear over-hung with grey clouds. You know how some evenings thick low clouds gather, black and angry clouds, even though no storm is approaching. Darkness and gloom descend before their proper time. The whole world makes you feel ill at ease, and all you want to do is to go and hide under the roof in a house made of bricks, skulk close to the fire with your family. (Solzhenitsyn, 1971, pp. 467–468) *Excerpt from* Cancer Ward *by Alexander Solzhenitsyn. English translation copyright © 1969 by the Bodley Head. Reprinted by permission of Farrar, Straus and Giroux, Inc., New York.*

When Solzhenitsyn writes of the '. . . herd instinct, the fear of remaining alone, outside the community . . .' he could be describing the *fear of philosophy*, the fear of resisting the easier answer, the fear of thinking for oneself. This fear is calmed by skulking close to accepted views, by adopting the opinions of others without making searching personal assessment, and by hiding behind verbal smokescreens. This fear is generated not only by the Russian social system, but apparently by all present functioning societies.

What Bacon says about the 'Idols of the Market-place' becomes obvious as soon as one makes a serious attempt to understand the meaning of words which do not have straightforward ostensive definitions. What becomes apparent is that these words have more than one meaning—these words have *meanings*.

Words can be Smokescreens

If we have only a vague idea of what we mean by a word, if we have only a hazy recognition of the possible range of meanings of a word but have never made the personal effort to clarify, then certain words can act a 'verbal smokescreens'. In Bacon's words they become 'barriers against understanding', making clear communication and full understanding impossible. Smokescreens can occur accidentally or be created deliberately by those who wish to conceal deeper issues—constant praise of the health service by some politicians might be an example of this—but the effect is the same: visibility is decreased, or even reduced to nil.

Raymond Williams and Keywords

Raymond Williams has explained that there are a number of words with which we are all familiar but which have more than one meaning. Not all words are of this type. We can agree about what is meant by words such as 'typewriter', 'library', or 'stethoscope', but some words, such as 'rationality', 'democracy', 'justice', and 'health', for instance, seem to be the source of continuing misunderstandings and disputes. Williams calls these words 'keywords'.

Williams regards his list, which is not comprehensive, as containing the words which play a major part in framing our experience of the world. He maintains that disputes over the correct meaning of these words can reveal the profound nature of the fundamental issues which underlie the words. But he also makes it clear that the substantive issues which exist behind the vocabulary cannot be understood simply by the analysis of words. He says:

> On the contrary, most of the real issues (remain) however complete the analysis, but most of them . . . (cannot) really be thought through, and some of them . . . cannot even be focused unless we are conscious of the words as elements of the problems. (Williams, 1976, p. 14)

In Williams's opinion the correct use of these words is not simply a matter of training. it is not a problem that can be solved by teaching an 'ignorant' pupil something that this quicker colleagues have learnt more easily. Perhaps the 'ignoramus' is not such a fool. It is not the case that one use of the word is correct and all the others are wrong. This mistaken belief is a brittle confidence—although unfortunately this confidence is not so brittle in practice, or newspapers and politicians would not be able repeatedly to shout of 'rights', 'freedom', 'democracy', and 'resolution' without a thought that they might be enshrining idiosyncrasy. Williams admits that if language is to be used at all it must depend upon the kind of confident attitude which believes that words have right meanings. If this was not so then everything would be permanently equivocal, and this would clearly be impractical, but the question of meaning must be faced, if only periodically. If it is not faced then the result can be a *false clarity of definition*—where once one definition has been selected from a number of possibilities that definition is insisted upon, thus screening the actual range of meanings, and the substantive issues, with an illusory clarity. For example, this screening can occur if it is insisted that health is simply a state in which no disease is present.

Examples of keywords

Democracy   One of the most confusing and abused words that Williams discusses is 'democracy'. It is so often used as a rhetorical bludgeon. Williams puts the problem succinctly:

> No questions are more difficult than those of *democracy*, in any of its central senses. Analysis of variation will not resolve them, though it may sometimes clarify them. To the positive opposed senses of the socialist and liberal traditions we have to add, in a century which unlike any other finds nearly all political movements claiming to stand for *democracy* or *real democracy*, innumerable conscious distortions: reduction of the concepts of *election, representation* and *mandate* to deliberate formalities or merely manipulated forms; reduction to the concept of *popular power*, or government in the *popular interest*, to nominal slogans covering the rule of a bureaucracy or an oligarchy. It would sometimes be easier to believe in democracy, or to stand for it, if the nineteenth century change had not happened and it were still an unfavourable and functional term. But that history has occurred, and the range of contemporary sense is its confused and still active record. (Williams, 1976, pp. 86–87)

Rationality   The words 'rational' and 'rationality' also have more than one meaning. In some cases these meanings are incompatible. The true nature of rationality is disputed, although most people agree that it is a characteristic that human beings should be proud of.

People can be described as rational if they are efficient in the pursuit of their chosen goals, or if they are logical, or if they are sensible, or if they are reasonable and realistic. There are also other legitimate meanings of rationality. The four meanings given above are, to varying degrees, different, but the main conflict can occur between the first two and the last two combinations—between a 'rational person' who is logical and efficient above all else, and a 'rational person' who is reasonable and sensible above all else.

It is not difficult to imagine cases where the different ideas of rationality clash, so that it becomes hard to say that both people are being rational. For instance, 'rational person A' might be pursuing the goal of bringing about political changes in a society which will deprive 80 per cent of the members of that society of all wealth, power, and voting rights. He might be pursuing this goal with great logic and efficiency— he might be a brilliant politician, logician, and legal expert. 'Rational person A' might be opposed by 'rational person B' who is trying to be fair and reasonable, and who is against the sort of ruthless extremism displayed by 'rational person A'. She might be concentrating on promoting the ideas of justice and of balance, and she may consider this to be the only rational course to take.

Are both people rational?

Gallie's Suggestion that all Legitimate Meanings of Words Must Share in an Historical Tradition

The philosopher of history, W. B. Gallie, has argued that certain 'concepts' (it is less confusing to substitute 'words' for 'concepts') are 'essentially contested'. His view, although similar to that of Williams, is not identical. Gallie says that there are some words about whose meaning people with different sets of values will never be able to agree. The meanings of these words must be sufficiently complex, ambiguous and adaptable to allow the formation of various schools of thought about their proper meaning. The meanings of these words must remain disputable in order that competing schools of thought can persist.

Gallie goes further than Williams. He claims that each 'concept' must possess some historically based core of meaning which is recognized as part of the 'concept' by all who use it. Without this there seems no reason why one cannot argue that a particular 'concept' can mean anything one wants it to mean—which clearly will not do. Gallie claims that each school of thought about the correct meaning of a word will agree about an 'exemplar'—an example of meaning which is not disputed. This exemplar will knit together and organize the main competing positions. There will be a tradition which links the various positions to a mutually respected common ancestor. Gallie says that:

> . . . the adequate understanding of such concepts involves some appreciation of their history. At the very least we must accept that every proper contestant use of such a concept can be traced back to a commonly acknowledged exemplar, and can be justified on the ground that, and to the extent that, people can be found who regard it and can rationally defend it as the best possible development of the original exemplar's aims. (Gallie, 1964, p. 189)

There is much in what Gallie says. In order to have any worthwhile conversation about the best meaning that a word has it must be possible for the debaters to have some common ground on which to base their discussion. For instance, in the case of democracy it might be agreed that all democrats must be egalitarians. In the case of art the debaters will be able to find a piece of work which they both agree is an example of art. And in the case of health they might be able to agree that health is essentially to do with wholeness. However, there are problems with Gallie's argument.

1. Words do not necessarily have undisputed meanings which can be traced back in history. As Williams has pointed out, meaning depends more on the ways in which a word is currently being used than on an appeal to some ancient ruling.
2. This means that Gallie's suggestion merely pushes the controversy back a degree. Instead of there being disputes about the legitimacy of particular meanings the arguments are centred on which is really the *true* exemplar. Williams comes nearer to the truth when he shows that words can often be used with a variety of meanings, *some of which may be contradictory*, without there necessarily being any point of agreement recognized by the protagonists. This does not rule out the possibility that there is a hidden common factor which does not conform to an ancient tradition.
3. In the case of the word 'health' Gallie's suggestion fails. Even though the idea of 'holistic medicine' is presently finding growing popularity, a great deal of 'health care' is still concerned with parts of people. Medicine pays attention to specific tissues, organs, and diseases in the name of health. Medicine is frequently not concerned with restoring people to 'wholeness', but with restoring them to a more limited idea of health. For instance, it may be enough for medicine to cure a disease in a person who before and after the treatment had other conditions which were not dealt with. In such cases medicine still claims to be working for health.

An Example of How Philosophy can Clarify Meaning

In the following section the words 'definition', 'theory', 'concept', and 'conceiving' are discussed. The meaning proposed for each can be contested.

It is important for a book on health to be clear about which meaning of each word is preferred because the words are used frequently in most writing about the nature of health. Usually this use is confused and confusing, but this need not be the case. Progress can be made on several fronts simultaneously.

Definition, theory, concept, conceiving

Definition   A definition is a specific, fixed label designed to indicate one meaning of a word or a phrase. A definition can be either a single word or a set of words. A definition is impersonal and must be communicable in language. Definitions are important in that they provide initial footholds towards understanding, but if they are thought to be 'the last word' then they are the foundations of dogma. Definitions can never be the 'last word' since all definitions must include theories, and theories change over time. The dividing line between definitions and theories is fuzzy.

Theory A theory is designed to explain more than a definition. A theory can be impersonal, it can be articulated publicly or it can be held privately. Theories aim for consistency internally and externally. That is, theories are designed not to be self-contradictory and to be consistent with features outside their own structure which they are designed to explain.

Karl Popper and Michael Polanyi agree that theories, formulated in language and made public, are no longer part of the inventors of those theories. Polanyi thinks that a theory on which a person relies is unaffected by any fluctuations which occur within that person. He says:

> A theory is something other than myself. It may be set out on paper as a system of rules . . . it is not I but the theory which is proved right or wrong when I use such knowledge . . . A theory cannot be led astray by my personal illusions. To find my way by a map I must perform the conscious act of map-reading and I may be deluded in the process, but *the map* cannot be deluded and remains right or wrong in itself, impersonally. (Polanyi, 1973, p. 4)

Theories are necessary for reasoned understanding and they allow practical changes to be made to the physical world. This is not the place to discuss the range and types of theory. The point to note is that it is possible to express theories independent of the theorist.

Concept Concepts are often thought to be very vague and nebulous. The 'concept of health' is supposed to contain many elements which all have something or other in common. People discuss 'cluster concepts' as if concepts were huge, rather shapeless, umbrellas sheltering some related ideas. Rock stars write, or used to write, 'concept albums' when they had a vague idea that they wished to explain something quite complicated through their music, or when all their songs seemed to have links. Used in these ways the word 'concept' is used to justify imprecision. The nature of health is not clear so health is referred to as a 'concept', but this is cowardice. It is ducking the issue. It is said that health is a 'cluster concept', and is many faceted, but this does not help us understand what we are thinking or what we are trying to do. To use the word 'concept' in this way actually imposes a convenient barrier to further thought and clarification. It is an excuse for sloppy thinking.

There is a better way of understanding the meaning of the word 'concept'.

Concepts must be held personally because they involve an essential personal element based on feeling, experience and memory. Concepts can be described externally although not without residue.

Personal concepts are unique, will be ambiguous and will contain various meanings. Concepts are not personal theories since they do not aim to be consistent, and involve more than theory. Theories might be part of personal concepts, and parts of concepts might be developed into impersonal theories.

Concepts are not innate in a person but develop as a result of interplay between conceiving, theory and practice. Concepts are not inherent in nature.

There is no such thing as *the* concept of health. Concepts are not 'out there', independent of human beings, waiting to be discovered. *The* concept of health is always either one particular theory of health or collection of theories of health whenever 'it' is referred to in the literature. *A* concept of health always refers to a particular articulated theory. What is meant when 'the/a concept of health as the absence of disease' is referred to is a crude *theory* that health involves the absence of disease. This has been put into words and so can be discussed, developed and perhaps tested in some way. It is not putting forward a concept to say that 'disease is a biological imbalance in a normally hierarchically harmonious arrangement of cells, tissues, and organs', it is the beginnings of a theory.

A concept cannot be fully articulated. A concept is held personally. A person's concept of health could involve the thought that disease must not be present, but it will involve more than this. It will involve *memory*, recollections of diseases experienced, of times when no disease was present (if this ever was the case), of happiness, of comfort, of waking up feeling that one could take on the world. Also it will involve the constant interplay between personal conceiving and changing circumstance. This personal element cannot be translated without residue. What a person feels and thinks about his concept can be described—although a lot must remain which cannot be put into words—at which point part of the concept will have become an articulated theory. The theory of a concept is never the same as the concept. It will probably have become considerably more consistent as a result of the translation.

A problem

Could a person possess a concept of health which made reference to anything he chose, however ridiculous? For instance, could a person possess a concept of health which involved the theories that health is undesirable, equivalent to suffering, that health is indicated by the colour blue, that health involves the creation of impediment, and so on? The person is clearly conceiving, and he may be on to something which will ultimately culminate in an impersonal theory. However, as it stands his concept is *impotent*, and this is an important distinction. To be powerful a concept must have *external relevance*. Other people must be able to understand what the concept means in theory or in practice, or both. Other people must be able to see the point of it. Not any collection of ideas counts as a concept of health because the potency of a concept depends upon an interplay between conceiving, consensus, articulation, illustration, and physical states of affairs. The sense of a potent concept must be able to be transmitted through theory and practice to other people. To be meaningful, to be more than a collection of unconnected individual ideas, a concept must have an identifiable focus or subject area.

Examples of concepts

In general, people's concepts of 'evolution' and 'mind' for instance, involve theories, examples, personal experience, analogy, imagination and personal puzzling, whether they realize it or not. Within each concept some of the theories may be internally inconsistent, and some may not be fully compatible with each other. The examples are drawn from such sources as discussions, books, and museums.

People's concepts of evolution, often in an incomplete and disorganized fashion, take account of Darwin's theory, neo-Darwinian variation of this theory, Creationist counter claims, gaps in the fossil record, theories of chance and determinism, personal opinions about plausibility, and so on. Similarly, people's concepts of mind might take account of theories about the nature of the brain and the correspondence between patterns of electrical activity and patterns of thought, behaviourism, personal experience of dreams, *déjà vu*, dualism, Descartes' thought, the 'soul', and religious implications amongst other things.

Even 'simple' concepts, such as concepts of colours, smells, sounds and so on, cannot be divorced from personal experience. I have an image of a red amaryllis but I cannot imagine red in the abstract. It is always a ribbon, or paint on canvas, or chalk on a wall, and so on.

Conceiving This is the capacity that people have which enables us to form concepts and theories. It permits choice, decision, and assessment. It is the basic ability by which we understand anything. The capacity can be revealed through conversation and through introspection, and does not require investigation by psychology to be apparent. Conceiving occurs frequently; conceiving is the act of assessing, weighing up, entertaining ideas, playing with inconsistencies, appealing to personal experience, fitting theories with perceived states of affairs, and inventing analogies. *Theorizing* is part of the act of conceiving but is more specific. Theorizing is directed towards the solution of immediate problems.

Arthur Koestler's book, *The Act of Creation*, gives a full and fascinating account of how this power of theorizing (which he believes is possessed by all sentient beings) provides solutions to problems for which no specific rules have been given. He argues that such situations are remarkably common. The key is not held only by people of exceptional genius who can somehow come up with an entirely new idea. This is mythical. The key to a new perspective is *synthesis*, and synthesis can take place only when thinkers are able to escape rigid rules to conceive more freely:

> When life presents us with a problem it will be attacked in accordance with the code of rules which enabled us to deal with similar problems in the past. These rules of the game range from manipulating sticks to operating with ideas, verbal concepts, visual forms, mathematical entities. When the same task is encountered under relatively unchanging conditions in a monotonous environment, the responses will become stereotyped, flexible skills will degenerate into rigid patterns, and the person will more and more resemble an automaton, governed by fixed habits, whose actions and ideas move in narrow grooves. He may be compared to an engine driver who must drive his train along fixed rails according to a fixed timetable.
>
> Vice versa, a changing, variable environment will tend to create flexible behaviour patterns with a high degree of adaptability to circumstances — the driver of a motor car has more degrees of freedom than the engine-driver. But novelty can be carried to a point — by life or in the laboratory — where the situation still resembles *in some respects* other situations encountered in the past, yet contains new features and complexities which make it impossible to solve the problem by the same rules of the game which were applied in those past situations. When this happens we say that the situation is *blocked* . . . A blocked situation increases the stress of the frustrated drive. What happens next is much the same in the chimpanzee's as in Archimedes' case.

When all hopeful attempts at solving the problem by traditional methods have been exhausted, thought runs round in circles in the blocked matrix like rats in a cage. Next, the matrix of organized, purposeful behaviour itself seems to go to pieces, and random trials make their appearance, accompanied by tantrums and attacks of despair—or by the distracted absent-mindedness of ... single-mindedness; for at this stage—the 'period of incubation'—the whole personality, down to the unverbalized and unconscious layers, has become saturated with the problem, so that on some level of the mind it remains active, even while attention is occupied in a quite different field ... until chance or intuition provides a link to quite a different matrix, which bears down vertically, so to speak, on the problem blocked in its old horizontal context, and the two previously separate matrices fuse ... The creative act is not an act of creation in the sense of the Old Testament. It does not create something out of nothing; it uncovers, selects, re-shuffles, combines, synthesizes already existing facts, ideas, faculties, skills. The more familiar the parts, the more striking the new whole. Man's knowledge of the changes of the tides and the phases of the moon is as old as his observation that apples fall to earth in the ripeness of time. Yet the combination of these and the other equally familiar data in Newton's theory of gravity changed mankind's outlook on the world. (Koestler, 1969, pp. 118–120. *Printed by permission of A. D. Peters & Co. Ltd*)

Theorizing is the process of choosing the most appropriate elements from one's concept of one or more subjects, refining, rejecting, and assessing for consistency, explanatory power, and simplicity. The forming of a theory is a personal activity which draws on the fullest range of human abilities. It is logically distinct from calculating, which is a process which can be specified precisely, and which machines can be programmed to do more efficiently than can people.

Personal conceiving is a prerequisite for defining and theory invention, and is ultimately necessary in order that decisions can be made as to the worth of competing theories. Conceiving transcends theory, paradox, and inconsistency. It permits judgement between theories without reliance on further theory. Conceiving allows a person to cope with the simultaneous existence of alternative and conflicting possibilities, whereas definitions and theories have a strictly limited focus. Conceiving is never static but is a liberating quality since it allows people to cope with change and unique situations.

Conceiving is not entirely language dependent but is also dependent on unspecifiable human factors which stem from experience of life. It is not the case that two human beings—who will inevitably have had different experiences—possessing knowledge of exactly the same theories will necessarily make the identical decisions in identical circumstances. Judgement is part of conceiving, and this aspect cannot be fully captured in words and symbols. The development of concepts and theories demands judgement at all stages, and this judging does not rest only on theory possession. It is not enough to know how to recite a theory, a person must know why he is reciting it, and what this means and implies.

The discussion of this section has shown how making the effort to clarify can be illuminating. Much present writing on health uses these words, often ambiguously, and sometimes with meanings different to those offered above. Whatever the case, knowledge of this clarification will enable a reader to understand more easily the intentions and thoughts of the various authors.

The results of the above clarification are used in Chapter Eight of this book.

Summary and Consolidation

1. This chapter has explained the extent of the problem of meaning. The problem is not only confined to discussions about health, but affects a wide range of keywords. The activity of philosophy can help dispel much of the confusion generated by the problem of meaning.

2. 'Health' is a word which is used with a variety of meanings. Which particular meaning is used seems, on the face of it, to depend on the context, the user, or both these factors.

Everyone involved with health in any way should attempt a personal clarification of the meaning of the word. Everyone should practise philosophy. It is not enough to read this book. The arguments and problems must be thought through and addressed personally.

3. Given that 'health' is a word which is used with a variety of meanings it should be possible to identify various schools of thought about its meaning. If the arguments of Williams and Gallie are correct then each school will understand health to have a particular meaning or range of meanings dependent on the values held by the members of that school.

4. In Gallie's opinion it should be possible to identify an historical tradition which links all the meanings preferred by current schools of thought to an initial exemplar. This is perhaps asking too much. However, it should be possible to discover a contemporary uncontested *general sense* of health—an idea which is an essential part of all the meanings of health and about which no-one would disagree. If the idea of health is not to be meaningless, if the word 'health' is not to mean anything one wants it to mean, then it must be possible to display some limit to the sense of the word.

Chapter Four
Theories of Health

Introduction

This chapter discusses four theories of health, and some of the ways of working to encourage health which are based on these theories. All the theories make sense when looked at from some perspectives, and each has inherent problems when seen in other lights. All the theories have been distilled and abstracted from much wider theories. This can create a rather over-simplified impression. However, the central points of each theory can be seen clearly and reflect the intentions of their authors accurately.

Clarification

Disease and illness

Before explaining the theories of health, something must be said about the words 'disease' and 'illness'. It will come as no surprise that these words are used with more than one meaning. Some initial clarification is essential.

It is not possible to define these words precisely, so that everyone will agree about their proper meaning, but it is possible to provide a fairly clear distinction between them although there is a persisting and substantial overlap. The professional philosopher Bernard Gert and Charles Culver, a physician, have collaborated to attempt a rigorous and analytical clarification of these and associated words. These writers are almost obsessive in their drive to uncover unequivocal definitions which can be used in practical situations. They worry that such important words are used too loosely at present:

> In the English language a cluster of words are used to refer to the conditions that concern us here. Three of the most important are 'disease', 'illness', and 'injury', but there are many more: 'wound', 'disorder', 'defect', 'affliction', 'lesion' and 'disfigurement', to list a few. While these terms have distinct though partly overlapping connotations, which can be fairly precisely identified, there is nevertheless an arbitrary element in the labelling of the various conditions . . . An interesting example of the arbitrary nature of this labelling is the condition experienced by deep sea divers who return from the depths too quickly. It is referred to as either 'caisson *disease*' or 'decompression *illness*', while essentially all of the associated ill effects are due to the cellular *injury* caused by nitrogen bubbles forming in the various bodily tissues. (Culver and Gert, 1982, p. 65)

In practice in medical science the identification of disease depends on measurement and comparison against normal states. Typically this process of identification evolves

26

from the description of a few unusual cases, to the description of a general 'disease pattern' (called a syndrome) for which the cause is not clear, to the description of a specific condition with a known cause. Early in the history of medicine the identification of disease, and the ways of distinguishing one disease from another, depended solely on the sorts of signs and symptoms reported and presented externally. As techniques developed the diagnosis and understanding of disease rested on the underlying tissue changes, and now hinges mainly on biochemical analysis. In each case what was and is described as a disease is a pattern of factors which have occurred in sufficient people for a specific type of deviation from a particular norm to be identified.

Throughout history any diagnosis of disease has assumed that a satisfactory definition of the word exists. According to Culver and Gert this assumption has not been justified. They discuss a number of past definitions of disease, and dismiss several as being woefully inadequate. For instance they find fault with a definition offered in William White's book, *The Meaning of Disease* (White, 1926). This is:

> Disease can only be that state of the organism that for the time being, at least, is fighting a losing game whether the battle be with temperature, water, micro-organisms, disappointment or what not. In any instance, it may be visualised as the reaction of the organism to some sort of energy impact, addition or deprivation. (White, 1926)

The authors conclude, bluntly and correctly, that on this definition one wrestler held down by another is suffering a disease. They also condemn a definition found in a standard pathology textbook as being far too general, vague and all inclusive. This definition is:

> Disease is any disturbance of the structure or function of the body or any of its parts; an imbalance between the individual and his environment; a lack of perfect health. (Peery and Miller, 1971)

Culver and Gert comment ruefully that this offers three separate, equally poor, definitions. Clipping nails, puberty, and being tied to a chair are all diseases according to the first definition! The second definition is too vague to be useful, and the third is circular. What it says is that having a disease is to lack perfect health, and that people lack perfect health when they have a disease. The question of what a disease is remains untouched.

Culver and Gert go on to discuss more acceptable definitions and prefer those which refer to *deviation from a norm for a species, biological disadvantage,* and *a medical disorder that is intrinsically associated with distress, disability, or certain types of disadvantage.* They offer their own definition of a 'malady' which incorporates the 'cluster of words' to which they refer. However, as far as a definition of disease is concerned they accept that put forward by Lester King which incorporates the notion of a range of evils, and also the idea that deviation from a norm is necessary:

> Disease is the aggregate of those conditions which, judged by the prevailing culture, are deemed painful, or disabling, and which at the same time, deviate from either the statistical norm or from some idealised status. (King, 1954, p. 197)

There are those who would find fault with this definition, since it contains the idea of illness as well as disease. The sociologist David Field has offered a useful partial separation of the terms. He argues that the word 'disease' refers to a medical conception of pathological abnormality which is indicated by a set of signs and symptoms. And 'illness' refers primarily to a person's 'ill-health' and is indicated by *feelings* of pain and discomfort. So diseases are indicated by signs that can be detected by medicine, and recognized as abnormal, and illnesses are subjective experiences of pain and discomfort. This means that illnesses can be the result of pathological abnormality, but need not necessarily be so. A person can feel ill without medical science being able to detect disease. For instance, a person can feel 'under the weather', be depressed, have no energy, be emotionally disturbed, be in pain, and be in despair, without recognized disease being present. Conversely, a person can have no symptoms of illness and yet be diseased. For example, cervical cancer can be detected by a Pap smear even though there are no subjectively experienced symptoms of discomfort, and teeth can decay without causing pain. Disease, on this account, is a measurable abnormality while illness is experienced as a quality. Human beings cannot measure their feelings in the same ways that they can measure physical states.

Field's distinction is part of an argument he puts forward against the blinkered nature of medicine. He thinks that since disease relates to the organic level (according to accepted modern characterization) and illness to the psychological and social level, by focusing almost total attention on disease scientific medicine does not pay as much heed as it should to all the aspects associated with sickness. For instance, a person's psychological reaction to his disease is often neglected. Consequently in some contexts, it can be detrimental to believe that diseases and illnesses can always be demarcated clearly because both disease and illness are events which happen to whole human beings. Some diseases/illnesses do not seem to fall neatly into one category or another. For instance, it is not clear whether alcoholism should be considered to be a disease or an illness. Nor is it obvious how to classify a person who has a significant allergy but no current symptoms.

Summary

Diseases can be thought of as certain sorts of abnormality that occur in parts of people's bodies. These abnormalities can be identified by medical science. Illnesses are feelings that people experience. It is important to make this distinction because 'disease' and 'illness' are words which are often used as if they are interchangeable, which is not always the case. People 'feel ill', they do not necessarily 'feel diseased'. A person cannot be ill without feeling it, but a person can be diseased without feeling it. A further distinction is that while some diseases can be infectious, illnesses cannot. Medicine works to control and eradicate disease. In so doing it can also be working to beat illness, but some illnesses, some aspects of ill-health, are not the province of medicine. These illnesses may have a range of causes against which medicine has no defence. If the words 'disease' and 'illness' are habitually conflated this makes the profession of medicine appear to have more power and scope than it actually has. It is useful to bear this in mind. It is an important clarification.

A simplified summary of theories of and approaches designed to increase health

Theories of Health

The theory that health is an ideal state:

—A 'Socratic' goal of perfect well-being in every respect.

—An end in itself.

—Disease, illness, handicap, and social problems must be absent.

The theory that health is the physical and mental fitness to do socialized daily tasks (i.e. to function normally in a person's own society):

—A means towards the end of normal social functioning.

—All disabling disease, illness and handicap must be absent.

The theory that health is a commodity which can be bought or given:

—The rationale which lies behind medical theory and practice.

—Usually an end for the provider, a means for the receiver.

—Health is lost in the presence of disease, illness, pain, malady. It might be restored piecemeal.

A group of theories which hold that health is a personal strength or ability—either physical, metaphysical or intellectual:

—These strengths and abilities are not commodities which can be given or purchased. Nor are they ideal states They are developed as personal tasks. They can be lost. They can be encouraged.

Approaches Designed to Increase Health

The sociological approach

—Concerned with a range of factors which influence health—for good or bad. Works to describe inequal distribution of disease and illness, and the inequal use of the Health Service by different sections of the community. Tries to explain the causes of these inequalities in terms of socio-economic, political, personal, environmental, biological and chance factors.

—Its findings are used to provoke changes in society.

The approach of medical science

—Emphasis on clinics, hospitals, biology, statistics, and measurement of conditions against normal standards.

—The causes of disease and the effects of drugs and surgical techniques are researched to increase understanding and to allow preventive, curative, and educational measures.

The humanist approach

—Regards health as a positive goal to be achieved personally. Disease, illness and other problems can co-exist with health.

—Recognizes that people are complex wholes living within, and permanently influenced by, a constantly changing world. Recognizes that there are interconnections between the physical, the spiritual, and the intellectual.

—Recognizes a latent ability for self-development in all human beings who have the actual or potential ability to understand the implications of their actions.

Common Factor

In general, the provision of the conditions necessary for the achievement of some biological and chosen potentials, and of conditions which enable people to work towards the achievement of other biological and chosen potentials is the goal of all approaches. Much of the provision of suitable conditions is achieved by the removal of obstacles.

The chart displays four distinct types of theory: the theory that health is an ideal state; the theory that health is a level of fitness necessary to perform the tasks expected of a normal person in a society; the theory that health is a commodity which may be bought or given, gained or lost; and the group of theories which hold that health is a personal strength or ability. The various types of theory have elements in common. For instance, to varying degrees disease, illness, handicap, and pain must all be absent in three of the four types of theory. Also all theories, except the theory that health is an ideal state can, again to varying degrees, be described as being both a means and an end. It is possible to devise compatible combinations of the theories. For example, the gaining of health thought of as a commodity could enable a person to function normally in society, this normal functioning could be seen as evidence of a personal strength and might also boost a person's ability to cope, and the combination of these states could be what the individual would describe as ideal. However, when these theories are examined in depth it is clear that, at other levels and in other contexts, they can also be incompatible. For instance, the theory that health is an ideal state is not necessarily consistent with that of health as being normal functioning in a society since most people would deny that their present function is ideal, indeed many would argue quite the opposite. Health as normal functioning is not necessarily consistent with the theory that health is strength since such strengths are often *created* at times when normal functioning is disrupted, and it is possible for strength to exist regardless of considerations about normal functioning. In addition, the theory that health is a commodity is, in many circumstances, actually *opposed* to health as strength since commodities are given or purchased and health as a strength or ability to respond positively can be seen as a personal task which requires *effort* to be achieved.

To some extent the theories are compatible, and to some extent they are not. Sometimes the theories and approaches aim at the same target, at other times they set their sights on different marks. However, the targets *are* set in the same metaphorical rifle-range.

The boxes shown on the chart are not fixed or watertight. People's thoughts about health are usually complex and can vary in different contexts. People do not usually have one set opinion about health, rather they draw on elements of different theories. Similarly, the various approaches designed to increase health do not make use of just one theory. People who adopt a particular approach can recognize the merits (and demerits) of other theories just as they can recognize the value of other approaches. The point of presenting such a simplified model of such a complicated area is the same as that of this whole book: to make things clearer so that we know where we stand, and to enable us better to identify the implications of each theory and approach if each is adopted in a particular practical context.

Theories of Health

The theory that health is an ideal state

Theories which hold that health is an ideal state, a state of supreme wellbeing, have always been a part of human dreams. Our own age is no exception. The World Health Organization offered this famous definition of health in its *Constitution* of 1946:

Health is a state of complete physical, mental and social well-being and not merely the absence of disease and infirmity.

In one important respect this definition is commendable. Its intention is to show that health involves more than not being infirm and not having a disease. The definition tries to focus attention on wider aspects of human life to show that health is something which is positive and enhancing, and is not achieved just by not being ill and diseased. The World Health Organization has been consistent and energetic in arguing and working to achieve their vision. The current ambition of the organization is *Health for All by the year 2000*. One of their primary goals is the cessation of all war by this date. Unless this and other necessary conditions can be achieved, what they mean by 'health for all' cannot possibly come about. The aims of the World Health Organization are admirable and yet hopelessly idealistic. The thinking is that the target might as well be set as high as possible; although it will not be achieved, the higher it is set the higher the actual achievement will be. The ambitions are noble but they are seriously undermined by the fact that the proper basis for them—rigorous theoretical clarification—has not been established. As it stands the definition and theory are little more than well-meaning rhetoric. Both are so comprehensive that they are almost meaningless.

What is wrong with this definition and the theory which inspires it?

1. Although the definition states correctly that health is more than the absence of disease and infirmity, it also assumes that a person cannot be healthy if she has any kind of physical or mental disease or illness, or if she has any kind of infirmity. It even assumes that a person cannot be healthy if he happens to be suffering from any kind of social problem. The definition describes health as an absolute, and so maintains that there is only one legitimate standard of health, but to set such a standard condemns most, and probably all, human beings to the disheartening belief that each of us is permanently unhealthy.
2. The definition does not face up to the many controversies about what is meant by the phrase '. . . complete physical, mental and social wellbeing . . .'. The meanings of the terms '. . . physical wellbeing . . .', '. . . social wellbeing . . .' and '. . . mental wellbeing . . .' are all disputed. The selection of the actual states to be described by such phrases always depends on the values of the people who are offering the descriptions. For example, social wellbeing in a kibbutz is a different state to social wellbeing in a new development of 'executive homes' in a leafy English suburb. In the suburb a person's state of social wellbeing could hinge on whether he possesses two cars or a mere one, whereas social wellbeing is achieved by sharing resources within the community in a kibbutz. Which condition is true social wellbeing? Which is the ideal? Similar difficulties are involved with the other phrases. For instance, in the USA an ambitious, successful, egoist business woman would probably be described as having mental wellbeing so long as she was content, but in Russia such a state of mind could, quite plausibly given the ethos of that social system, be taken as a mark of a sickness.

There is a further problem for the World Health Organization to face if it wishes to see its theory of health become a practical reality. What counts as mental wellbeing is contested by people who have different views about what the phrase means. It is quite possible for a person to put forward an argument that their mental wellbeing depends on their being able to write and to distribute racist literature. If the person found such activity fulfilling and it made him happy it would be difficult to argue that his practice did not contribute to his mental wellbeing. The trouble is that (a) not everyone will agree that the racist author and publisher actually does have mental wellbeing, and (b) the activities of the person could certainly harm the mental wellbeing of other people. Consequently, if 'health for all' means that every member of the human race must have mental wellbeing then 'health for all' will never be achieved whilst the mental wellbeing of different individuals is in conflict.

3.   The third problem is that although it may be an inspiration for some to have such a supreme and idealistic, personal and global, goal to aim at, it can mislead other people into striving for something which cannot possibly be attained. This can deflect some people from more realistic goals and lines of development and achievement. Rene Dubos (1959) has explained, in an influential early work on the nature of health, that the theory that ideal health is possible is a mirage which continues to draw people on, but which is of no help in leading humanity to a real oasis. Dubos's argument is that contemporary dreamers either refer back to an imagined past utopian era in which 'ideal health' was universally achieved, or look forward to a future utopian goal. He says that what he calls 'tribal memories' can become transmuted into mythical recollections of idyllic happiness experienced in a 'golden age', and that the future vision for our generation is offered by what he calls 'the magic bullets of medicine'. It is often thought that if only the right treatment for our ills could be found, if only real 'miracle drugs' would become available, 'ideal health' could be reclaimed, or achieved at last. Dubos argues that this is a myth which seriously distorts the true nature of health.

4.   To talk of 'ideal health' as if it is an absolute, specifiable, definable state is a mistake. It is as meaningless and useless as asking for a description of a perfect human being. What would such a person be like? Would such a person be male or female; five, twenty or sixty-five; black, white or yellow; an athlete, an intellectual, a comedian; a miner, a poet or a bank manager? The point is that people have different bodies, ages, backgrounds, and talents. The optimum state of existence for different people is bound to be different in each case.

5.   There is a sense in which an individual can have a personal ideal state which could be described as full health. Such a state would probably be experienced only fleetingly. However, there is another sense in which it is not possible for any person to have 'ideal health'. This is if health is thought of as the maximum fulfilment of all the potentials of a particular individual. Such a state cannot be achieved because all human beings possess more latent potentials than they can ever fulfil. Choices are made throughout a person's life about which direction to take, about which potential to develop and about which potentials will have to lie dormant. At school choices are made about whether to specialize in maths, technology, science, the arts, or art and design. Such specialization continues to be forced on people because life is short. Much potential has to remain untapped.

Some latent potentials cannot be realized at the same time because they would be in conflict. For example, an obsessive pursuit of business goals would leave no room for voluntary work overseas, although both potentials could once have been latent in an individual simultaneously.

The implications of applying this theory   There is little more that can be said about the implications of this theory. It is cast in such a general way that it impresses at first sight, and there is no doubt that the motives which lie behind it are laudable, but if the question of how it is to be put to work is pursued it becomes clear that it is impractical for a number of reasons.

The theory that health is the physical and mental fitness to perform socialized daily tasks

The American sociologist Talcott Parsons advocates this theory. In Parsons' opinion health is:

> . . . the state of optimum *capacity* of an individual for the effective role and tasks for which he has been socialized. (Parsons, 1981, p. 69)

This definition is part of a wider theory about the way in which society functions. This theory is too complicated to be discussed properly here. This is not a great disadvantage since his theory of health makes sense removed from the wider context. Parsons's idea about health is that the word means the standard of physical and mental function necessary for a person to perform the activities which are expected of him, according to the norms of the society in which he lives. At first sight this does seem to be a plausible way of thinking about health, so long as one is content to regard health and disease as opposites: people who are diseased or ill are often unable to continue normally. Of course, having a disease need not be the only reason for this. Nor need it be the end of the story. If an alternative account of health is preferred the deliberate refusal or inability, to continue normally need not be a sign of mental or physical illness but of a 'healthy' desire for change.

According to this theory of health a person cannot be described as healthy if she has a *disabling* disease or illness. Parsons does not consider the possibility of degrees of health. He states quite plainly that health is an *optimum capacity*, so anything less than this cannot be what Parsons calls health.

If a person is no longer able to function normally he will, according to Parsons, adopt the 'sick role'. If individuals adopt this role, they can claim the right to be excused from their normal social duties, but are also obliged to seek the medical advice of friends, relatives, and healers because they have a duty to get better.

What is wrong with this theory?

1. It describes health in terms that are too narrow. Health is conceived as the polar opposite of disease and illness. It is disease and illness which interfere with a person's capacity to perform the tasks for which he has been socialized. But health is more than the antithesis of disease and illness. Theories which fail to recognize this are inadequate.

2. The theory is unappealing to those, such as the World Health Organization, who regard health positively. Parsons' theory is neutral in the sense that it sees health as a state which must be achieved in order to continue as before, rather than being associated with positive change and improvement in people's lives. The theory does make sense when applied to individuals who are happy with their lives, who enjoy their work, and who are achieving and developing along ways of their choosing, but it falls down in cases where the '. . . role and tasks for which he has been socialized . . .' are not stimulating for a person. The role and tasks might even be part of a counter-productive process. It can be that working in a physically or mentally stressful, or monotonous, job—or never having worked at all—is precisely that which causes individuals to adopt the 'sick-role' in the first place. For illustrations consider the work of miners, workers on building sites, and business people working long hours under high levels of stress. Miners often develop diseases of the lung as a result of years of exposure to coal dust; tradesmen and labourers in physically demanding jobs are often injured and they tend to 'burn out' as their physical strength fades with age, and business people can suffer such problems as excessive drinking, and heart disease at an early age as a result of their jobs. In cases such as these advocates of this theory must face a very tricky question. It is this: how does it make sense for a person to work for, or be assisted towards, a return to a state of health (that is, the state of optimum capacity of an individual for the effective role and tasks for which he has been socialized) when that state will inevitably eventually contribute to a state which will be described as ill-health according to this theory?

The implication of applying this theory To work for health in this sense is to work to maintain societies in their present states.

The theory that health is a commodity

The predominant image which overshadows medicine and the British health service is that health is a commodity. That it is something—albeit an amorphous thing—which can be supplied. Equally, it is something which can be lost.

Why talk of health as if it were a commodity? What is meant by such a phrase? According to this way of looking at life health can be given or purchased without personal involvement in the process. For example, 'medical health' can be purchased by buying surgery or drugs to cure a person's heart disease. The use of a drug gives health. The drug brings health with it. Health is seen as somehow substantial. It seems to be a nebulous entity which can be gained and lost. Health appears to be a thing which exists apart from people, which may be captured if the right procedure is followed. This sort of health can be lost if a person has a diseased organ, but with appropriate treatment it can be restored piecemeal.

Health as a commodity is a belief which has stemmed directly from the approach of medical science. It is thought by those who see health in clinical terms that individuals are somehow naturally healthy, and would remain healthy if it were not for some untoward outside influence creating a physical problem. Given normal luck and normal circumstances people are healthy but just as a person can lose a wallet so a person can lose health if abnormal circumstances obtain.

To sum up, there are two main elements to the theory that health is a commodity. Firstly health is thought to be a commodity *apart* from individuals (something which can be given via drugs, for instance), and secondly, at times, health is thought of as an ideal goal which can be recaptured given the right sort of medical intervention. These two themes combine in subtle ways.

What is wrong with this theory?

There is a sense in which the theory is very plausible. Certain conditions have to be fulfilled, certain things have to be provided, in order to create some aspects of health. Some of the commodities offered by medicine can improve health.

However, what concerns the opponents of this theory is the very idea that health can be thought of as a commodity, as a commercial object. Oliver Sacks, a neurologist and practising physician, is strongly opposed to the idea. Sacks shares many of the opinions of the humanists. In common with Dubos he acknowledges that the approach of medical science, from which the idea of health as a commodity sprang, has advantages, but that this approach is not sufficient to solve all the problems encountered in working to increase health. Sacks claims that being a true physician requires the ability to combine the pursuit of science and the pursuit of art harmoniously. He believes that being a physician is a 'romantic science'—a vocation which needs general laws, algorithms, procedures, and mechanisms, but which also requires empathy, communication at a personal level, non-verbal understanding, and the intuitive art of emotional interaction. Sacks rejects the idea of health as a commodity because it ignores the art required of a physician—after all, he argues, a machine can dispense drugs and information—and because it ignores the fact that human beings are unique and incredibly complex wholes. The approach of medical science, the approach which nurtured the notion of health as a commodity, has much to offer but it must be viewed in a proper, balanced perspective. Sacks says:

> . . . we pretend that modern medicine is a rational science, all facts, no nonsense, and just what it seems. But we have only to tap its glossy veneer for it to split wide open, and reveal to us its roots and foundations, its old dark heart of mysticism, magic and myth . . .
>
> There is, of course, an ordinary medicine, an everyday medicine, humdrum, prosaic, a medicine for stubbed toes, quinsies, bunions and boils; but all of us entertain the idea of *another* sort of medicine, of a wholly different kind: something deeper, older, extraordinary, almost sacred, which will restore to us our lost health and wholeness, and give us a sense of perfect well-being.
>
> For all of us have a basic intuitive feeling that once we *were* whole and well; at ease, at peace, at home in the world; totally united with the grounds of being; and that we lost this primal, happy, innocent state, and fell into our present sickness and suffering. We had something of infinite beauty and preciousness—and we lost it; we spend our lives searching for what we have lost; and one day, perhaps, we will suddenly find it, and this will be the miracle, the millennium. (Sacks, 1982, pp. 26–27)

Sacks believes that the search for our 'lost health' through the acquisition of commodities is an illusion which has sometimes been encouraged by the apothecary or physician. Sacks sees health as a personal fulfilment, whether a person's chosen goal is happiness, a sense of reality, a feeling of being fully alive, or whatever is personally fulfilling, but health is not the achievement of some blissful ideal by collecting commodities. What Sacks describes as 'this basic metaphysical truth', that health is a personal fulfilment, can be:

> . . . suddenly twisted (and replaced by a fantastic, mechanical corruption or falsehood). The chimerical concept which now takes its place is one of the delusions of vitalism or materialism, the notion that 'health', 'well-being', 'happiness', etc. can be reduced to certain 'factors' or 'elements'—principles, fluids, humours, commodities—*things* which can be measured and weighed, bought and sold. Health, thus conceived, is reduced to a *level*, something to be titrated or topped up in a mechanical way. Metaphysics in itself makes no such reductions: its terms are those of organisation or design. The fraudulent reduction comes from alchemists, witchdoctors, and their modern equivalents, and from patients who long *at all costs* to be well. It is from this debased metaphysics that there arises the notion of a mystical substance, a miraculous drug, something which will assuage all our hungers and ills . . . (Sacks, 1982, p. 28)

A central point against the theory that health is a commodity which emerges from Sacks' passionate appraisal is that by seeking to offer health only as a commodity, and by holding out the false hope of an effortless return to 'ideal health', the approach of medical science conceals from people their wider potentials because it undermines their unique 'metaphysical' (spiritual and intellectual) strengths.

The implications of applying the theory are discussed in a later section where criticisms of the approach of medical science are considered.

The Group of Theories which Hold that Health is a Personal Strength or Ability

This group of theories can be united under a general humanist banner. It is ultimately immaterial to the humanist view of health whether or not a person is diseased, ill, or suffering. Sometimes these states are necessary in order to allow an individual to grow, although in general the humanist recognizes these states to be obstacles which should be removed if possible. It is accepted that people can be helped to develop themselves by the removal of impediment by any means, including the means offered by the approach of medical science.

As we saw from Sacks's criticism of the theory that health is a commodity, it is insufficient to regard health only as a commodity to be dispensed piecemeal. Instead, this group of theories puts forward the view that health is either an unquantifiable resilience or an ability to adapt positively to the inevitable problems and sufferings that life throws up—it is not something which goes in the presence of disease and illness and returns with their passing. Health is a way of *responding* appropriately, and not only in biological ways.

Health is thus a means towards further and greater ends—if a person can resist or adapt positively to problems of different kinds then she has a position from which she can develop her potential to the full. Of course, this strength and ability to adapt positively can often be a significant and difficult end to be achieved in itself. This group of theories recalls the position of two hundred years ago where health was thought of only in holistic terms. According to these theories health is, once again, not something which can be precisely defined. It is a way of living—a 'whole rule of life'.

The Theory that Health is a Metaphysical Strength—the View of Oliver Sacks

It is important to understand the unusual experiences which have shaped Sacks's deeply held beliefs. Otherwise it will not be clear why Sacks believes with such passionate conviction in the existence of a deep unquantifiable human strength.

Sacks claims to have witnessed an awesome 'spiritual health' in his work with patients suffering from an array of debilitating mental and physical handicaps. He has described many bizarre, frightening, and yet inspiring case histories of a fascinating group of patients in *Awakenings* (Sacks, 1982). His book is important for several reasons. The most compelling of these is that it is possible to conclude that despite enduring the most extreme disabilities Sacks's patients fought back however they could: their human spirit could not be drowned in spite of everything. The great tragedy is (although Sacks does not make this explicit) that this spirit can be totally concealed in many normal individuals living in normal societies.

The theme of Sacks's book is to describe the lives and reactions of the few survivors of 'the great sleeping-sickness epidemic' (encephalitis lethargica) of sixty years ago, and at the same time show the implications of their struggles. Of particular interest is how the patients responded to the so-called 'miracle-drug' L-DOPA (*laevo-dihydroxyphenylalanine*). The euphoric reaction to the arrival and promise of this drug incited Sacks to a vehement attack on 'medical magic'. Although the immediate effects of L-DOPA were often dramatic, 'awakening' many people from years of immobility, the drug failed to restore sufferers permanently, and often caused worse illness than the original disease—although on balance Sacks feels that L-DOPA should be described as beneficial.

Sacks explains that the 1916–17 winter in Vienna saw the start of a 'new' disease which spread worldwide over the next three years. At a very rough estimate five million people died or were ravaged by the sickness. No two patients ever manifested the same picture. The most frequently occurring set of symptoms was somnolent illness which was followed by Parkinsonian effects (Parkinson's disease is a syndrome of symptoms with 'festination' prominent. Sufferers will experience hurriedness of steps, movements, words, and thoughts, with the feeling that this hurry is not caused by their own volition). Sacks states that a viral cause was eventually identified.

The pandemic raged for ten years to disappear in 1927. A fairly common pattern was that a sufferer would experience severe, comatose, sleep or equally severe insomnia, but that after a period of time, whilst the virus was still at large, a sufferer could recover to some extent only to experience Parkinsonian effects. Sacks states that over a third of the sufferers died during the initial stage of the sleeping sickness, either in states of coma so deep as to preclude arousal, or in states of sleeplessness so intense as to preclude sedation.

> Patients who suffered but survived an extremely severe somnolent/insomniac attack of this kind often failed to recover their original aliveness. They would be conscious and aware—yet not be fully awake; they would sit motionless and speechless all day

in their chairs, totally lacking energy, impetus, initiative, motive, appetite, affect or desire; they registered what went on about them with profound indifference. They neither conveyed nor felt the feeling of life; they were insubstantial as ghosts, and as passive as zombies. They were . . . awaiting an awakening which came (for the tiny fraction who survived) fifty years later. (Sacks, 1982, pp. 14-15)

Sacks points out that approximately 500 'positive' disorders have been noted. Among the most common he lists *akinesia* (total lack of movement — the inability to make voluntary movements), *aphonia* (the inability to make sounds), *aphrenia* (the stoppage of thought), and *akathisia* (the inability to keep still, an intense urge to move, restlessness or fidgets to a most extreme degree). Some patients could be 'living statues' for days and even for years on end. Some could speak, some:

. . . showed automatic compliance or 'obedience', maintaining (indefinitely and apparently without effort) any posture in which they were put or found themselves, or 'echoing' words, phrases, thoughts, perceptions or actions in an unvarying circular way . . . Other patients showed disorders of a precisely antithetical kind . . . immediately preventing or countermanding any suggested or intended action, speech or thought: in the severest cases, 'block' of this type could cause a virtual obliteration of all behaviour and also all mental processes — such constrained catatonic patients . . . could suddenly burst out of their immobilized states into violent movements or frenzies . . . (Sacks, 1982, p. 17)

Patients also displayed a wide spectrum of 'tics' (spasmodic twitches of the facial muscles) and compulsive movements at every functional level — yawning, coughing, sniffing, gasping, panting, breath-holding, staring, glancing, bellowing, yelling, and cursing. Nearly half the survivors became liable to extraordinary 'crises', in which they might experience such effects as an almost instantaneous attack of Parkinsonian symptoms, catatonia, tics, obsessions, hallucinations, 'block', increased suggestibility or negativism, or even a simultaneous combination of these disorders. These crises would last for a few minutes to hours before disappearing as suddenly as they had appeared.

The point of explaining a little of the detail of these unfortunate people's great suffering is to give an idea of the extent of their disability which none the less could not completely hide their spirit, desires, and potentials from a man of Sacks's obvious sensitivity. He was frequently overwhelmed by the impression of a tremendous inner strength in his patients which even the most severe difficulties could not extinguish. He makes the case that this spirit is not a product of his imagination, or a manifestation of the illness, but a quality which actually exists and which drives people to continue to develop in the face of apparently insurmountable odds.

'Miriam H.' is a patient of Sacks who during her long illness has suffered violent furies, apathetic depression, and crises in which she was morose and was compelled to look up at the ceiling. Miriam was partially paralysed and chair-ridden. She was given three courses of L-DOPA and always responded well at first, but twice had to have the treatment discontinued because of the occurrence of severe crises. Her third treatment was a relative success in so far as she learnt to control her crises and showed 'a clear-cut if unspectacular therapeutic response'. He writes of her:

. . . all in all, Miss H. has done well — amazingly so, considering the existence she has led.

Against all odds, Miss H. has always managed to be a real *person* and to face reality without denial or madness. *She draws on a strength unfathomable to me, a health which is deeper than the depth of her illness.* [Second set of italics added.] (Sacks, 1982, p. 128)

The theory that health is a reserve of physical and mental strength

The group of theories which hold that health is a personal strength or ability has received support from recent sociological inquiries into the 'health beliefs' of 'ordinary people'. Separate researches into 'lay concepts of health' have produced evidence which indicates that health is sometimes thought of as a reserve or stock of strength. Such a view of health is held by people of at least distinct cultures (by elderly Aberdonians, by Mexican peasants, and by middle-class Parisians). For instance, Mexican peasants were found to speak of people with a 'stock of health' as possessing '*sangre fuerte*' (strong blood) whilst a study of elderly Aberdonians showed that people with 'reserves of health' were believed to be able to withstand bouts of illness, but people who had 'lost their health' were considered to be 'done' or 'washed out'. They would have no energy left, and would be 'fading away'.

Rory Williams, the social scientist who studied the Aberdonians, found that the elderly people he interviewed felt that 'health' could be lost completely or partially, but might be recovered, and that 'weakness', the opposite of 'health', was another state which might develop. This weakness need not be a disease. It is more a proneness to be ill. The interviewees could be accused of some illogic, and of having notions that are not well thought through, but the central theme stands up. The idea that health is strength is one that has a real meaning for people, and not merely a meaning which has been constructed by academics. Williams writes:

> That health is something more than the absence of disease has been suggested by the notion of good health as the power of overcoming disease which is actually present. To this may . . . be added the complementary notion of bad health as the loss of such power even when disease is absent. (Williams, 1983, p. 192)

Williams' report shows that 'lay-people', not surprisingly, think of themselves as wholes:

> . . . though health is thus sometimes the absence of serious disease, it is also possible to refer to someone as healthy even though serious disease is said in the same breath to be present.
>
> The meaning of this conjunction of health or strength with disease was most clearly illuminated by my informants in accounting for a severe crisis which had been surmounted and which had ultimately proved transitory. A brother was described as 'the strong one of the family': his leg was amputated because of gangrene, he was put into 'this sort of glasshouse they put you in', he actually died and was resuscitated, and though he was never expected to come up out of this illness — he did. People who were well, strong, fit or healthy had the power to 'come through' or 'come up'; and hence they could also declare that they had always been healthy despite a list of sicknesses and diseases which was often alarming.
>
> Hence although health can be used simply to mean the absence of disease, it is also used in a far more complex and positive sense; and this positive sense often

dominated discussion by my samples of the relation of health to activity and moral effort. (Williams, 1983, p. 189)

The theory that health is an ability to adapt

This theory has obvious links with the other two in this group, and draws on points already discussed, but it also has its own identity. Versions of this theory have been put forward by writers such as Katherine Mansfield, Rene Dubos and Ivan Illich (Mansfield, 1977; Dubos, 1959; Illich, 1977).

Dubos and Illich argue that the influence of medical science should be less because *it impedes people's abilities to adapt autonomously*. Part of their case is that it is not exact laboratory science that has developed the most effective techniques by which to avoid disease and illness. Improved health (meaning here a decrease in the prevalence of disease) has arisen mainly as the result of social measures designed to correct the ills of industrialization, to provide better nutrition, better housing and better work conditions. The practical achievements of the nineteenth-century reformers did not come from an understanding of the medical problems. Laboratory science advanced understanding by discovering the complex world of germs and nutrient balances, but the practical improvements came as a direct result of improved hygiene and sanitation. Dubos writes:

> The time has passed when explorers on land or at sea have to depend on heavy loads of lemons and animal food in order to protect themselves against scurvy and other deficiency diseases. A few small packets of synthetic vitamins can now make an adequate diet out of proteins, carbohydrates, fats, and water. A dash of chlorine and an effective filtration bed will make any water supply more typhoidproof than the most sparkling streams brought from high mountains . . .
> But while modern science can boast of so many startling achievements in the health fields, its role has not been so unique and its effectiveness so complete as is commonly claimed. In reality . . . the monstrous spectre of infection had become but an enfeebled shadow of its former self by the time serums, vaccines, and drugs became available to combat microbes. Indeed, many of the most terrifying microbial diseases — leprosy, plague, typhus, and the sweating sickness, for example, had all but disappeared from Europe long before the advent of germ theory. (Dubos, 1959, p. 19)

Dubos goes on to make the point that other maladies, such as cancer, vascular disorder, and mental disease, which were not affected by the sanitary movement, remain as problems. He suggests that the causes of these ills may be directly related to modern life (he implicates pollution and excessive competition) which does not allow man sufficient time in which to adapt.

Dubos's argument is cast against the utopian theory that health is an ideal state for all people. He points out that such a utopia cannot be achieved because of the constantly changing nature of existence, and such a state should not be desired because human beings are so adaptable that they can live and flourish in almost any Earth environment. A utopia is static and real life is not like this. Dubos claims that the capacity to explore and create and face the dangers and challenges of new environments is an essential human characteristic, and that to define one way of life alone as 'healthy' (which is a possible consequence of an arrogant interpretation of abstract general definitions of health) is a form of dictatorship. Such an esoteric interpretation could act to confine the human spirit, which should be free.

Dubos thinks that health should be thought of in very wide terms which permit scope for differences of opinion. This is why he has opted for a theory of health which states that health is equivalent to the ability to adapt. He does have faith that the scientific method has the potential to discover the causes of all disease, and to suggest remedial procedures, but this is not the whole story of health. He says:

> Whether concerned with particular dangers to be overcome or with specific requirements to be satisfied, all the separate problems of human health [Dubos seems to mean disease here] can and eventually will find their solution. But solving problems of disease is not the same thing as creating health and happiness . . . Health and happiness are expressions of the manner in which the individual responds and adapts to the challenges that he meets in everyday life. And these challenges are not only those arising from the external world, physical and social, since the most compelling factors of the environment, those most commonly involved in the causation of disease, are the goals that the individual sets for himself, often without regard for biological necessity. Nor can the problem be usefully stated [sic] by advocating a return to nature . . . Harmonious equilibrium is an abstract concept with a Platonic beauty but lacking in the flesh and blood of life. It fails, in particular, to convey the creative emergent quality of human existence . . . The Garden of Eden, the Promised Land that each generation imagines anew in its dreams, and all the Arcadias past and future could be sites of lasting health and happiness only if mankind were to remain static in a stable environment. But in the world of reality places change and man also changes. Furthermore, his self-imposed striving for ever-new distant goals makes his fate even more unpredictable than that of other living things. For this reason health and happiness cannot be absolute and permanent values, however careful the social and medical planning. Biological success in all its manifestations is a measure of fitness, and fitness requires never-ending efforts of adaptation to the total environment which is ever-changing. (Dubos, 1959, pp. 22-25)

Dubos's argument that health is an ability to adapt recognizes that health is not an absolute, specific, uncontroversial end in itself. It is not a permanent, definable target for which successive generations of human beings, whatever their circumstances, can strive. For Dubos health is an ability to respond positively to the different challenges which arise in people's lives.

What is wrong with this group of theories?

1. They are all too vague. The natures of the strengths and abilities referred to are not specified. It is not clear what the 'metaphysical strength' discussed by Sacks is, nor is it obvious what a person's 'reserve of strength' is. The meaning of the phrase 'health is the ability to adapt' seems straightforward at first sight, but no clear details are given about what the possession of such an ability involves. In all cases nebulous non-physical qualities are being offered as partial descriptions of the true nature of health.

   The issues have not been pressed far enough by the various authors. They are all satisfied with their answers after having turned over only the top spit of soil. To provide an adequate theory of health it is necessary to dig deeper and not to accept fine sounding words because they are euphonic.

The theory that health is the ability to adapt provides the best illustration of how this group of theories falters. The problem is, once again, that without a comprehensive study of 'nutrition', 'one man's meat is another man's poison'. It is not possible to reach universal agreement about what a 'positive adaptation' to the ever-changing world is. Unless the theorists who hold that health is an ability to adapt give more substance to their theories, unless they give reasons why such views as these are mistaken, it will often remain quite legitimate to argue that such responses as insanity, larceny, suicide, murder, megalomania, and apathetic depression are positive adaptations to external circumstances. They are certainly adaptations, and if they can be justified by some as being positive then in the absence of a comprehensive list of approved inclusions and exclusions they must count as positive examples.

2.   Because of this vagueness, because of this sugar-coating of ambiguity, people who wish to work for health are given no concrete targets at which to aim, and few guidelines about how to achieve these targets if they do exist! In order to increase health, whether it is thought of as strength or as the ability to adapt, health workers must have a fair idea about the types of element which make up the strengths and abilities so that they can be encouraged in those people who lack them.

If such strengths and abilities are innate then this too should be clearly explained, if only to save health workers the trouble of wasting their energies on fruitless tasks. If this is the case then health workers would be released to do work which has a real practical benefit.

The implications of applying this group of theories

If the elements of people's lives which are relevant to their reserves of strength and their abilities to adapt could be specified more clearly, then the implications for practical health work would be great. The current vogue of regarding medical care and health care as synonymous would pass out of fashion to be replaced by the idea that it is people's abilities to cope and to take full charge of their own lives that are the most important features of work for health. Instead of maintaining health centres staffed almost entirely by medics and para-medics, such places would offer a far more comprehensive service. They would, for instance, focus on how people in the same families can have different non-physical strengths and abilities. From this sort of study health centres could try to devise ways of helping everyone to achieve a higher standard.

However, without more details of the natures of such strengths and abilities no-one can be sure who the best professionals for the work would be, or if they should be professionals at all. Would increases in people's strengths and abilities to cope be best served by psychologists, teachers of social theory, teachers of economic theory, psychiatrists, nurses, medics, solicitors, teachers of basic maths and English, counsellors, members of various churches, politicians, philosophers, or some other group? More precise theories are required before the implications for practice can be worked out.

Approaches Designed to Increase Health

The sociological approach

Social scientists of various sorts produce much valuable research which shows that a person's class, work, and standard and style of living can affect his life span and the sorts and severity of disease and illness which he is likely to suffer in his lifetime. *Inequalities in Health: The Black Report* (Black, 1982), written by a group chaired by Sir Douglas Black, President of the Royal College of Physicians, provides extensive information about the ways in which class differences are associated with differences in 'health'. This, and a host of similar research reported regularly in such journals as *Social Science and Medicine*, indicates that people's chances of avoiding such diverse problems as back pain, injury, depression, diabetes, epilepsy, bronchitis, kidney disease, heart disease, and cancer improve according to the quality of their class. There is a demonstrable connection between levels of illness and social position.

Problems

Social research is vital. It produces a stream of information which argues for itself that the world's social systems, to differing degrees, do not treat a great number of people fairly, that injustice can produce physical and mental problems, and that things could clearly be better. But the approaches joined under the broad banner of 'the sociological approach' suffer from these problems:

1. There has been insufficient analysis of the meanings and sense of the word 'health', and not enough notice taken of the scope of the various theories of health. Ample evidence of this can be found in most sociological journals concerned with medicine, illness, and health.
2. This means that although sociologists constantly point out that health is much more than just a target for medicine, and that if it is true that diseases are suffered more commonly by people of lower classes then health is naturally and inevitably a political issue, they have not made the further step of acknowledging that health is more than the opposite of disease and illness. To put the issue very crudely, many sociologists think in terms of a continuum such as this:

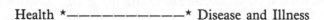

Health *––––––––––* Disease and Illness

where health is achieved when disease and illness are absent. In common with the badly misnamed health service, sociology is still primarily concerned with the causes of illness and disease—believing that if all of these could be eliminated then full health would follow—than it is with the question of what health really is and how this can be achieved. A recent book by Jeanette Mitchell, *What Is To Be Done About Illness and Health?* (Mitchell, 1984) is fairly typical in this respect. The author asks such questions as: What is the nature of the connection between the work we do, the money we earn, where we live, how often we get sick, and the kinds of illnesses we suffer? Where do the chronic illnesses, heart attacks, cancers, and handicaps come from? Why do some people get them and others not? How can we account for the present pattern of illness and death, with its stark class contrasts? Is all this illness inevitable? What is the medical system doing to remedy the problems we face? Could medicine and health be different?

She then offers interesting and informative answers to these questions. She makes the point that:

> There could be less chronic and recurrent illness. Our problems are less a matter of biology than politics. Better health is possible. (Mitchell, 1984, p. 41)

The fact which emerges clearly from her writing is that, whilst she recognizes that health is a wide-ranging issue influenced by many factors and of interest to many diverse professions, she cannot let go of the simplistic equation that not being ill must be the same as being healthy. She points out that the now classic definition of health offered by the World Health Organization is rather mystical, but she does not think that the issue has to be complicated. She says:

> But what we want is not really hard to grasp. We want fewer chronic and recurrent illnesses, less cancer and heart disease, less depression and anxiety. Of course we cannot hope to abolish illness, but the important point about the class pattern of health and illness . . . is that it is evidence of how much unnecessary ill health most people face. The level of health presently enjoyed by the people at the top of British society should not be seen as an absolute standard, but it is at least an indicator of how much better our health could be if our lives were different . . . the top civil servants [have] a quarter the rate of heart attacks of men at the bottom of the Whitehall hierarchy; [there is] twice the level of chronic illness among people in social class five compared with social class one; levels of chronic depression among working-class women [are] five-times greater than among middle-class women. That's a lot of unnecessary illness we could do without. (Mitchell, 1984, 213–214)

This writer, and social science in general, is concerned with a major aspect of the problem of how to achieve health. Social science has shown that membership of social classes 4 and 5 is an obstacle in itself, and can create further unnecessary obstacles such as disease and illness. By displaying the problem social science works to remedy it, but this is not the full story. Social science fails to acknowledge that a person can be ill, diseased or handicapped and yet still enjoy a reasonable degree of health.

3. A consequence of these two problems—that the meanings of health are not fully discussed and understood, and that health is equated with the absence of illness and disease—is that much social science has the appearance of being thoroughly predictable to observers both within and outside the discipline. A common reaction is that Marxist sociologist X and Functionalist sociologist Y and Methodological Individualist sociologist Z have all discovered the same new horse to ride. Each either assumes that the nature of health is known or initially defines it in a way which will suit her conclusions. And each naturally believes that the social system and social theories which they advocate are best equipped to provide the maximum possible health.

Health has become the issue of the day and offers a splendid opportunity to produce the old arguments in different clothes. There is some truth in this opinion. Consequently the results of social research have less of an impact than they should. Much disturbing information lies buried to a wider audience.

The approach of medical science

Western medicine espouses a scientific approach which is designed to increase health thought of in a particular way. The approach of medical science has a number of clearly identifiable features. Many of these are problematic and have been the subject of widespread criticism in recent years. These criticisms have not, on the whole, been digested by the medical establishment, but it is true that not all medics endorse the following generalized views of medical science.

Assumptions of medical science

1. *That health occurs when disease is absent.*

2. *That health is a commodity.*

The medical approach favours the theory that health is a commodity. This idea is encouraged by the medical industry which supplies the drugs and the technology. It has been argued that the purpose of medicine within a market economy is primarily to match this supply with a demand which medicine is partially responsible for creating. In a recent book, André Gorz makes the point that:

> Fundamentally . . . *the practice of medicine is a business.* The relations between medical professionals and the public are market relations. The professional sells what the patients ask for or are willing to buy *individually.* (Gorz, 1983, p. 186)

Inequalities in individual health are explained by pointing out that different social groups have unequal access to medical products. This sort of thinking furthers the myth that society has a supply of health locked away which needs only to be tapped, processed, and then sold; and that the medical industry has products which are directly responsible for increases in health. It is still commonly believed that increases in the quantity of the 'health supply' (drugs and implements) are bound to lead to corresponding increases in the levels of health of individual people.

3. *That medical science has produced a body of certain knowledge which can be applied to bodies as bodies rather than bodies as people.*

4. *That the best way to cure disease is to reduce bodies to their smallest constituent parts.*

Bodies are thought to be complicated biochemical machines. It is believed that there is an unbroken chain of cause and effect in physical disease which can best be attacked at its most fundamental level. This outlook means that molecular and electrochemical disturbances and abnormalities have become the main point of focus for medicine, and that other influences on people are paid less attention. It also means that it is thought that the 'certain knowledge' can be applied impartially to all sets of molecules, without regard to the person or to the person's interaction with the world.

5.   *That health can be quantified in relation to norms for populations, particular groups of individuals, and individuals.*

6.   *That medicine is and should be a form of engineering.*

It is assumed that a doctor can separate himself from his subject just as an engineer can when he is maintaining a bridge. It is further assumed that the maintenance of health is a matter of technical proficiency—that the doctor can ensure normal functioning by keeping tissues and molecules in their correct order.

Problems

Medical science does help people overcome a range of physical difficulties, but the discipline must also take heed of the criticisms that have been made of it.

1.   Medical education and practice is predominantly concerned with the structure and function of the body, and with disease processes. Medicine is practised mainly in hospitals and clinics. Although medicine does instigate epidemiological research it does not pay sufficient attention to the wider social and economic causes of disease and illness which have been identified by social scientific research. The best ways of dealing with disease and illness are not necessarily those which concentrate primarily on curing existing biochemical abnormalities.
2.   Medical science disregards the unquantifiable aspects of people. It treats the emotions and spirits of human beings as mostly irrelevant to medical practice. This demeans people.
3.   Medical science argues that full objectivity is possible—that doctors can be totally detached from their patients. Work in the philosophy of science has shown that this degree of objectivity is not possible, and that medical scientists are not as removed from their subjects as some of them believe (see the Appendix for a more complete discussion of this point).
4.   The idea that health can be quantified can, according to some medical thinking, be translated into the definition that *health is the normal state of individuals and populations*. This emphasis on quantification has its advantages. Statistics and measurement provide a sharp focus and gauge for practical treatment and care. There are a great many features of individuals and populations that can be measured. For example it is possible to measure the level of haemoglobin in a person or groups of people; the average number of children per family; the major sources and amounts of protein in the diet of a population; the height, mobility, and speech of a child at a certain age; the life expectancy of men and women, and so on. These features can be surveyed and the results analysed in order to calculate the particular 'normal condition'. If this norm is not being achieved by an individual, or by groups of individuals within populations, then steps may be taken to try to ensure that the situation improves.

What is worrying about this definition is that, taken on its own as *the* criterion of health it can act to justify an existing state of affairs which would, on other standards, be described as undesirable. This definition of health implies that the normal standard, whatever this may be, is desirable when this need not be universally agreed. The normal 'state of health' of groups of children, or a single child, in a village in the Third World and the normal 'state of health' of groups of children, or a single child, in 'suburban Britain' might differ drastically. Which children are healthy?

Work in the sociology of medicine heightens this worry. A theme in this discipline is that health is often used as a normative term. It is claimed that health is socially defined and so is achieved when a person does not deviate physically, mentally, or behaviourally from certain norms which can vary over time and between societies. If this is so then it can be legitimately argued that both groups of children, those in the Third World and those in Britain, are healthy, but is this an acceptable conclusion? Which is the true norm? Is it one or the other, or is there a third alternative?

Consider these cases: the history of medicine records that the haemoglobin levels of young women in a Victorian workhouse were measured and an average calculated. This quantified norm was then assumed to be the correct standard of health, but this was in fact a poor standard. The haemoglobin levels of the women were so low that they suffered from chlorosis (a form of anaemia in which the skin takes on a greenish colouration), but since they had been defined as healthy their peculiar skin colour and lack of energy was explained as being a normal physiological condition of young women during puberty. To take another case, where are the 'norms of health' to be set for unique individuals? A mentally retarded child might be achieving certain expected norms, but this achievement could distract all attention away from her other abnormal abilities. She might, for instance, have latent artistic talent which will never be tapped because of her otherwise satisfactory performance.

The main point which stands out from this problem is that other criteria and considerations are essential if the definition *health is the normal state of individuals and populations* is to be used.

The foremost critic of medicine in recent years is the theologian Ivan Illich. His criticisms of the medical establishment pose further problems for the approach of medical science. They are not all entirely valid but none of them should be ignored.

Ivan Illich's case against medicine

Illich is a radical opponent of medical science. He believes that the practice of modern medicine has, for a number of reasons, created new types of disease. He writes:

> The medical establishment has become a major threat to health. The disabling impact of professional control over medicine has reached the proportions of an epidemic. (Illich, 1977, p. 11)

Illich insists that for the most part medicine is itself a major impediment to the achievement of health. He discusses *iatrogenesis*, by which he means diseases, sufferings or obstacles actually created by medical intervention:

> Increasing and irreparable damage accompanies present industrial expansion in all sectors. In medicine this damage appears as iatrogenesis. Iatrogenesis is clinical when pain, sickness and death result from medical care; it is social when health policies reinforce an industrial organisation that generates ill-health; it is cultural and symbolic when medically sponsored behaviour and delusions restrict the vital autonomy of people by undermining their competence in growing up, caring for each other, and ageing, or when medical intervention cripples personal responses to pain, disability, impairment, anguish and death. (Illich, 1977, p. 271)

Illich provides substantial lists of the 'harmful side effects' of many drugs, and of 'unnecessary surgery'. He argues that surgery and chemotherapy are actually new forms of epidemic and that scientific medicine has made all of us patients. We are now so subordinate to medicine that the essence of our humanity, our autonomy, is seriously threatened. Now that the more fatal epidemics have disappeared modern medicine has set about creating its own. According to Illich, medicine must do this in order to remain as an instrument for the bureaucratic control of societies.

Medicine has thus not only harmed health in the sense that it has created illness and disease, but it has also harmed health in the sense that it has decreased autonomy. In Illich's opinion there has been a total 'medicalization of life' in the West. This has had a disabling effect, undermining a basic humanistic principle—the principle of self-determination. Illich's invective makes the most sense when what he means by health is understood. Illich thinks that:

> Health designates a process of adaptation. It is not the result of instinct, but of an autonomous yet culturally shaped reaction to socially created reality. It designates the ability to adapt to changing environments, to growing up and ageing, to healing when damaged, to suffering, and to the peaceful expectation of death. Health embraces the future as well, and therefore includes anguish and the inner resources to live with it . . . Health is a task, and as such is not comparable to the physiological balance of the beasts. Success in this personal task is in large part the result of self-awareness, self-discipline, and inner resources by which each person regulates his own daily rhythm and actions, his diet and his sexual activity. (Illich, 1977, pp. 273–274)

Illich's point is that conscious, rather than merely biological, adaptation is an essential part of being a person. Health is a process of adaptation which is dependent on personal autonomy. Autonomy itself is not health, but it is necessary for health. Autonomy cannot be given since it depends in part on personal qualities and energies, but it can be prevented if a person is placed in a situation where, for instance, he cannot choose his response because, through ignorance, he is in no position to do so. Seen in this light, Illich is saying that not all medical intervention creates disease and suffering, although a lot of it does, but professional medical intervention is inevitably, by its very nature, a counter to autonomy.

Illich regards the 'medicalization of life' as part of the general counter-productivity of an over-industrialized society (this is a theme which he has explored in other contexts such as education and energy utilization). Illich believes that the harm which is caused by this counter-productivity is a political harm since it involves a loss of autonomy. He argues that it follows that a political solution is required. In the case of medicine this means that individuals must reassert personal control over their own health.

In other words people must be allowed to adapt freely, which means that medical interference must be kept to a minimum.

Illich is insistent that:

> Thoughtful public discussion of the iatrogenic pandemic, beginning with an insistence upon the demystification of all medical matters, will not be dangerous to the commonweal. Indeed what is dangerous is a passive public that has come to rely on superficial medical house-cleanings. The crisis in medicine could allow the layman effectively to reclaim his own control over medical perception, classification and decision making. The laicization of the Aesculapian temple could lead to the delegitimizing of the basic religious tenets of modern medicine to which industrial societies, from the left to the right, now subscribe . . . the layman and not the physician has the potential perspective and effective power to stop the current iatrogenic epidemic. (Illich, 1977, p. 12)

Illich's optimistic position is that a number of individuals will somehow be able to convince the medics and the medical industry that the existing medical establishment will have to be dismantled. He explains that the present 'medical nemesis' is experienced by people who are 'largely deprived of any autonomous ability to cope with nature, neighbours, and dreams, and who are technically maintained within environmental, social and symbolic systems' — in other words people who are trained to fit neatly into society's slots. These lay-people will have to acquire the knowledge and the competence to evaluate the impact of medicine on health, and it is only the medical establishment which can make this possible.

Much of what Illich has to say makes sense. His criticisms should be read by all consumers and providers of medicine, but such a noisy polemic as the one Illich offers can cover up gaps which have not been thought through or filled by reasoned argument. Much of his research into the various forms of iatrogenesis is extensive and impressive and has not been refuted, but what he says about medicine is too black and white. The following points can be made against Illich:

1. There is not necessarily such a direct link between people lacking autonomy and the practice of medical science as that which Illich insists on. There are other reasons why people are not autonomous and do not develop their potentials. It is by no means inconceivable that medical science and the actual practice of medicine can enhance autonomy. Medicine can be used to relieve problems which would otherwise act against individual autonomy. Autonomy is affected if an individual has to spend his time caring for and trying cure himself, or if his problem limits the activities he would like to do in normal circumstances.

   Illich gives medical science little credit. Antibiotics can be used to control infection and need not always be used unwisely. Pain relief has become sophisticated, and not all surgery is unnecessary. For instance hip-replacement operations and heart bypass surgery can be most enabling. Also, the understanding of the causes of disease has undeniably increased.

2. Is Illich's vision realistic? How can the changes he suggests be made to come about? He does not tell us. In his discussion of the problems caused by medicine he does not cover the full reality of the situation. He does not propose a solution from 'where we are now', but from a point at which it would be conceivable

for things to change quickly. There are external influences which are bound to affect autonomy, such as traditions of behaviour, pollution, and corporate competition, which cannot be altered by autonomous individuals. In order to bring about the sweeping changes which Illich recommends people must come together in groups—collective action is necessary, but to join a group inevitably means sacrificing some autonomy in order to achieve the collective goals.

Illich gives little indication of the form his proposed 'self-care' should take. In one sense this is precisely his point—specifications and rule-following are anathema to autonomy. However, he also says that people whose lives have been 'medicalized' are 'largely deprived of any autonomous ability to cope with nature, neighbours, and dreams, and are technically maintained within environmental, social and symbolic systems'. And if this is the case then reasoned personal strategies are needed to enable people to deal with their environments and social pressures. Most people, as they are in the real world now, need at least some guidelines in order to begin to gain the confidence to adapt autonomously.

At times Illich seems to be advocating a return to the 'golden age' which his mentor Dubos has shown to be both impossible to achieve and not desirable to aspire to or to have if it were possible.

Witness these quotes:

> Famine will increase until the trend towards capital-intensive food production by the poor for the rich has been replaced by a new kind of labour intensive, regional, rural autonomy. (Illich, 1977, p. 266)
>
> A world of optimal and widespread health is obviously a world of minimal and only occasional medical intervention. (Illich, 1977, p. 274)

This is not obvious at all.

3. Although Illich argues that care should be done to oneself and occur within families he neglects the significant number of cases in which neither of these forms of care are possible. Young children, many elderly, the congenitally handicapped, the mentally ill, some accident victims, people with degenerative diseases (such as multiple sclerosis), the terminally ill, and others, are unable to care for themselves and often cannot be cared for within families. They may not have families, and if they do it will be the case that the autonomy of the carer will become subservient to the maintenance of the sufferer—an unsatisfactory state of affairs on Illich's own account. For such cases as these there is a need for a system of welfare (which would have to be professionally based) which does not place a total burden on individuals and families who are already suffering severely. Admittedly this welfare system need not rest on medical foundations, but, given the existing state of affairs and the possible natures of the problems of the sufferers, it seems highly unlikely that medicine would be out of bounds.

In sum, Illich's main difficulty is that shared by all those who advocate versions of the theory that health is an ability to adapt. He does not address the question of what this ability to adapt is, nor does he discuss how such an ability can be created and enhanced.

The humanist approach

Humanism is a label which can cover a range of theories. There is no single doctrine which can fully demarcate humanism. It is better to think of humanism as an attitude — as a way of living and believing. There is a fluid set of themes in humanist thought which are shared by humanists, although some humanists would include more themes in this set than others.

Humanism will never be characterized in exactly the same way by any humanist. For me humanism is an outlook which holds that the common interests of individual human beings are of primary importance and should take preference over the particular interests of individuals and groups. The humanist view is that all policies, whether scientific, medical, social, political, industrial or some other should take full account of the unique abilities of human beings to make reasoned choices, and to work to develop themselves. Humanism is opposed to the type of thought which believes that single solutions can be found which will apply universally to the ever-changing problems of human life. Humanism resists and counteracts dogmatism, and it stands against the propagation of 'blind knowledge'. Humanism acknowledges that practical knowledge is necessary for many tasks but it condemns in all cases the sort of 'education' which prefers training people to follow only given procedures rather than enabling them to think for themselves. Humanism challenges the view that people ought to follow policies which someone else has decided are in their best interests if the individuals concerned have not been given the information necessary for them to make their own judgements.

The most basic humanist position is that human dignity depends upon self-determination. This capacity for free choice is the source of morality: without the possibility of choice there is no possibility of morality. As a consequence humanism does not lay down hard and fast specific moral rules. A humanist has faith in his fellow human beings. The belief is that with increased autonomy people will come to recognize and respect the potentials that other human beings have: the recognition of the fullness of one's own humanity will generate a heightened feeling for the humanity and common interests of others. When stated in the abstract such dictums as do not do unto others what you would not wish for yourself, 'the rightness or wrongness of an action depends on the effect of that action on the welfare of all human beings', or 'act so that the effect of your action is compatible with the permanence of genuine human life' can appear to be nothing more than well-meaning platitudes, and certainly there are many instances where the practical application of such general guides is highly debatable and fraught with controversy. However, this does not detract from the overall worth of such ideals. It is a humanist theme that such maxims, once personally thought through, should be heeded whenever significant decisions have to be taken.

With respect to health humanism offers the view that health is a personal goal which people should be free to strive for by their own efforts. Humanists are convinced that all human beings possess a latent ability to develop themselves, so long as they have the actual or potential ability to understand the implications of their actions. Humanism never treats people as objects, as medical science sometimes has a tendency to do. Instead it is believed that people are incredibly complex physical, emotional, intellectual, and spiritual wholes (where 'spiritual' is used to mean having spirit rather than in a religious sense). No man is an island. A person cannot be considered in full if she is thought of in total isolation from the world. Such abstraction is not really possible. All people live within, influence and are permanently influenced by, a constantly changing world.

Since health is personal, health can be a different state for different people. According to the humanist account it makes little sense to think of health as an absolute, and since health is a personal task which all people, whatever their status, have a right to work towards, then it becomes correct to think that disease, illness, and other problems can co-exist with health. For instance, a cancer sufferer is diseased and is likely to remain so, but other legitimate health goals can still be set. It could be that the man has been bitter and selfish all his life, but has regretted his feelings. Now that he has perhaps all the more reason to feel these emotions he sets himself a new target of selflessness, contentment and kindness. If he achieves this target then he can justifiably state that he is healthy even though he might wish that he were healthier still.

A very important part of the humanist view is that self-development must be moral. It must be moral in the broad and general sense that if a person does not wish the consequences that his self-development has for other people to happen to him, then he must not develop himself in that way.

Problems

Many tomes have been written in praise of humanism, and there are humanist journals which try to apply humanist principles to practical problems. But in the case of health the changes in society that are needed to bring about the humanist notion of it are so great that the debate usually takes place on a 'worthy' yet very theoretical plane. What is needed is generally agreed. We need mutual tolerance and respect, a tolerance of other people's beliefs and customs, an awareness that other people have needs which are similar to our own, and we need an environment where people can choose and are then able to develop themselves in accord with their choices. The problem is that how these goals are to be achieved is not certain and so the discussion frequently hovers around the issue of what is the fundamental need. Opinion varies as to whether this is more and better education for all, the removal of class divisions, the provision of full employment, the undermining of personal ego, de-industrialization, de-bureaucratization, the elimination of nationalism, or the general increase in material prosperity, amongst other candidates.

What is needed is more earthy controversy. What is needed is a full theory of health which takes account of all that is good in humanism, and which puts forward concrete proposals. Inevitably these proposals will not be acceptable to all, but it is essential that they are aired in the arena of practice. If they are wrong, or too woolly, then they must be shown to be wrong or woolly. That all ideas should be exposed to the fullest possible criticism is another humanist theme.

Note: The Christian approach has not been debated in this book because, with the obvious difference, that humanism is not a religious doctrine, this approach shares many of the same prejudices as humanism.

The Common Factor

A number of key points have emerged or have solidified in this chapter.

1. *Health is not a word that has a single uncontroversial meaning.* Health does not have a core meaning waiting to be discovered. There is no undisputed example of health. This has been demonstrated by the fact that different theories of health exist which are all legitimate and plausible, but which regard health in different and conflicting ways.

2. *Health can be seen as a means or as an end.* Health can be regarded as an end in itself. This end can be different dependent on age, ability, circumstance, and so on. Health can also be seen as a means—a state which must be achieved in order that further ends can also be achieved. In many cases the achievement of the means can be a significant end in itself.

   Inevitably there are tapestry-like overlaps associated with this distinction, but this does not make attempts at segregation in appropriate contexts invalid since this can be an important aid to clarification. When factors that have been temporarily separated merge and combine in different ways at least we have a clearer idea about which elements are coming together. In many cases health can be described as either a means or an end depending upon the point of view of the person who is giving the description. For instance a medic could claim that by curing a specific disease in a person she has restored that person to health, but the patient may still have to spend time adjusting and convalescing—he might have lost a job or his friends through his disease. The patient may see the doctor's work as a beginning, as a means which will allow him to return to normal life eventually. This process will require more of the patient than just being free from disease.

   It is useful to know that there are two ways of viewing the goal of health. It can be important to point out to a person that what he sees as an end (perhaps it is his own physical wellbeing) is actually also a means by which he can begin to move in other directions. Perhaps he might go on to attempt personal intellectual growth, or he might choose to help others achieve their own physical wellbeing.

3. *People cannot be fully understood in isolation from what they do in their lives. Also people cannot be fully understood in only biological terms.* People have a great range of facets. Because of this diversity it is inevitable that the specialist approaches designed to increase health which focus on particular aspects will have different priorities and goals.

4. *Although there are some conflicts between the various theories and approaches there is a significant common factor.* This common factor is, on the face of it, blindingly simple, but on analysis the idea soon becomes plagued with difficulties. All the theories and approaches share an underlying sense even though they take health to have different meanings. This sense has to be cast in general terms.

   It is that *all theories of health and all approaches designed to increase health are intended to advise against, to prevent the creation of, or to remove, obstacles to the achievement of human potential. These obstacles may be biological, environmental, societal, familial, or personal.*

This states clearly that work for health is bound to be diverse. For example, in the cause of health a surgeon will operate to remove a tumour in order to give the organ or organs affected by the growth of the tumour the chance to achieve the potential it or they would have if not restricted by the tumour — which can be thought of as a *liability*. Another example of an attempt to remove obstacles to normal functioning is when a physician prescribes antibiotics in order to allow the body to continue its development unimpaired by unbeneficial influences. This work may also enable people to fulfil other potentials in their lives.

Social workers, health visitors, and politicians work to remove different obstacles to the achievement of potential. For instance, they may try to eliminate problems such as lack of heating, damp conditions, marital trouble, child abuse, unemployment, or poor employment. Such impediments may cause further impediment such as disease and illness, and they act in their own right to divert time and energy from avenues along which to achieve more important potentials. In yet another way professional health educators advise against practices thought likely to create obstacles, and they explain how a change in practice might help to remove existing obstacles. Educators of all kinds will try to explain how, in various contexts, people's potentials can be realized more effectively.

The elimination or prevention of obstacles is by no means only a negative operation. Elimination and prevention of obstacles to potential does not only involve cutting away. The removal of impediment can often be achieved only through addition. Obstacles can be created by such disabling factors as ignorance, cultural deprivation, insufficiently developed powers of conceiving, apathy, lack of hope, lack of competence, and lack of confidence. Such impediments can be remedied only by positive measures of change and addition. For instance, it is important, in order to eliminate certain obstacles, to provide more information and also more time to allow people to learn how to use and adapt this information to their own circumstances. And it is important to change environments, or social structures, or power possession, or prevailing attitudes and atmospheres, in order to provide more opportunity for people to begin to develop themselves. In order to remove many obstacles to achievement it is necessary to provide the right conditions for human flourishing.

The major point that is now clear is that issues of health are not only issues of disease and medicine. Health topics are inextricably linked with wider issues, issues about how people can and ought to conduct their lives. For many people it is the way in which a person is able to live that is the essential difference between health and ill health, regardless of bodily fortune or ill-luck. It is only for those convinced by mechanistic theories that health is a separate issue from personal life. Katherine Mansfield knew this well. She wrote:

> By health I mean the power to live a full, adult, living, breathing life in close contact with what I love — the earth and the wonders thereof — the sea — the sun, all that we mean when we speak of the external world. I want to enter into it, to be part of it, to live in it, to learn from it, to lose all that is superficial and acquired in me and to become a conscious, direct human being. I want, by understanding myself, to understand others. I want to be all that I am capable of becoming so that I may be . . . *a child of the sun* . . . But warm, eager, living life — to be rooted in life — to learn, to desire to know, to feel, to think, to act. That is what I want. And nothing less. That is what I must try for. (Mansfield, 1977, pp. 278-279)

When extracted from her passionate prose, Mansfield's definition of health is *the power to achieve*. Hers is a more poetic version of the more rigorous and analytic theory put forward in the next chapter.

An objection

It is time that the devil had an advocate.

> So far we have been led by the hand through several apparently plausible stages. We realize that there is a real problem about stating clearly whether or not a person is healthy, and we know that words can be used ambiguously. We see that there is a need to clear things up in the health field, and we recognize that there can be different theories of health, all of which have their problems. We are also prepared to accept that a very common factor in health work is the removal of different obstacles to different human potentials. But now we are being manoeuvred into accepting the truth of a further position *that a person's state of health cannot realistically be separated from a person's quality of life*. We have reached a point where we are no longer being coaxed. We are being led by the nose. We wish to go no further.
>
> There are several protests we could make, but one basic objection may be enough to show that the argument has already gone too far. It is that there has been too much playing with words—too many liberties have been taken. Most of the theories and approaches discussed stretch the meaning of the word health too far in order to suit their particular purposes, and the idea that *good health is equivalent to a good quality of life* has stretched meaning beyond breaking point.
>
> In reality health is a much more narrow topic than has been argued. Most of the theories of health, and most of the uses of the word health, are wrong. The British health service is correctly named. The health service pays attention to diseases and illnesses for the single purpose of restoring people to health. Health is the speciality of the health service. Other disciplines which claim to have an interest in health are merely tinkering. Health is a state which exists at one end of a continuum and has disease as its opposite, like this:
>
> HEALTH—————————DISEASE
>
> Health and disease are personal states to be enjoyed or to be suffered. There are various states in between, such as becoming ill and getting better.

Response

The objection is mistaken. It can be shown to be so without question.

Only in a limited sense does the present health service work to restore health. This point cannot be made too often.

1. An inspection of any etymological dictionary will show that the meaning of a word is not fixed once and for all, and that one word can be used with several different meanings. The meanings of words do change, but there are always limits which it is important to clarify.

    A controversial contemporary example of how the meanings of words can evolve accompanies the present information technology revolution. Prior to the invention of electronic computers the word *intelligence* was correctly applied only to living organisms, and then almost exclusively to man and the higher mammals. Now that computers can perform numerous complicated calculations at almost the speed of light, be programmed to design intricate blueprints, be programmed to program themselves, and be programmed to beat top-class human chess players, it has become widely accepted that it is correct to talk of *intelligent machines*. There are people who find serious fault with this practice, but they are in the minority, and their dislike of the new use of the word *intelligent* does not alter the fact that it is used meaningfully.

2. There are alternative views about health other than the medical model. These views actually have more in common with the idea of *wholeness*, which is the historical meaning of health. These alternative views are legitimate. They can complement and also conflict with the more limited medical view. Health can be thought of as an ability to fulfil a role, as a strength, and as an ability to adapt to changing circumstances. All views share a common sense which is wider than the limited meaning which has been officially adopted by the health service.

3. Even if health is thought to be a state which is the opposite of disease, even if this most limited meaning is chosen, then, because there are many and varied causes of disease and illness, wider factors than individual physiology and biochemistry must be taken into account. Social researchers such as Black, Mitchell, and Doyal have produced a wealth of evidence which shows that such factors as living conditions, work, economic policies, stress, and different sorts of pollution can cause disease and illness.

4. Present work within the health service is already wider than the idea of health put forward by the medical model. Many practising health educators and promoters, nurses, health visitors, counsellors, chaplains, and doctors try to help a person as a whole to cope with life as a whole. They work to help with such problems as finance and benefits, with housing and home helps, with sorting out future options for people, and they also often look to help the close family and relatives of their patients. All this is already done in the name of health.

5. Health is not an absolute. Health is not a fixed state. The optimum states that different people can achieve are inevitably different. Optimum states for single individuals are also different at different times in their lives. It is therefore mistaken to think of a static continuum such as the one presented above.

The idea that health is a specific, definable, fully describable state to which everyone can aspire equally is nonsense. It is as meaningless as the idea that there can be a perfect person. What would such a being be like?

Individuals are occasionally described as perfect by people whose faculties of reason are temporarily clouded by romantic mists. A 'Mr' or a 'Mrs Right' sometimes rides into a person's life. They are not, of course, everyone's choice of candidate for a perfect human being. The issue of health is similar. People are different—they have different ages, abilities, intelligences, disabilities, environments, ambitions, stresses, jobs, and so on. Health for a geriatric is not health for the runner Steve Cram. The health that Steve Cram enjoys might be thought to be marvellous health for a geriatric, but this misses the point. A geriatric could not possibly attain the physical state of a world record breaking athlete, although other aspects of her life could be better than Cram's.

Chapter Five
The Fullest Sense of Health

Review

This is a natural point at which to take full stock of the book so far. It is time to pause and to take a very deep breath before assessing an original and provocative theory of health.

What ground has been covered so far? What forward progress has been made? Looking back over the previous chapters what has become apparent is that there is no simple answer to the question 'What is Health?' The idea that health is desirable, that it is a 'good thing' to have, and that this is all that can really be said on the subject is not good enough. Different people have different ideas about health which can often be justified. Because of this they will naturally disagree about whether Dennis and the other case studies are healthy or not. People from different backgrounds who have different sets and orderings of values can, quite legitimately, mean different things when they speak of health. This is frustrating. One naturally expects commonly used words to have clear definitions, but what is most disturbing is that the various groups of professionals who seek to provide health are not yet fully clear about what it is that they are trying to do.

The problem of how to be clear about the meaning of health was left in the air for a while, during which time it was explained that there is, in general, a real problem about the meaning of words. This problem is by no means exclusive to the word 'health'. It is a significant problem which can affect the majority of human communications for the worse. Its existence must be acknowledged, and we must constantly attempt to deal with it. The way to tackle the problem of meaning is through philosophy. Philosophy is a clarifying process; it is a process which digs to the taproots of problems.

In the previous chapter various theories about health were assessed. Each tries to answer the question 'What is Health?' in its own way. None of the theories is fully compatible with any other, so they cannot be combined into one comprehensive theory of health. All of the theories are well-intentioned in their own ways, but each creates further puzzles. For example, precisely what is ideal health? How can this target be specified? How can health be equivalent to being able to fulfil a social role if that role is making a person unhappy? If health is strength how can we work to create this strength? Is it the most that we can do to bow to fate—to shrug our shoulders and say 'well, that's the way he's made'? How can we define the difference between positive and negative adaptation to changing circumstances? Dying after being run over by a bus is a form of adaptation—so is suicide, so is wife-beating, so is alcoholism, and so is safe-breaking. Arguably all these practices are debilitating. How can these be clearly distinguished from adaptations which enhance lives?

What is the next step? Can we abandon the problem here? Should we accept that health is an idea that is to be contested forever? Can we leave it that the limits of its meaning can ebb, flow, and bend at the whim of any new theorist, however crazy or clever, who claims to have discovered what health is really about? We have discovered that all theories about health and all approaches which are designed to improve health do share at least one element in common. They may ascribe different meanings to the word 'health' but they agree, implicitly at least, that work for health is work towards the removal of obstacles of many kinds which face people in their lives. This is progress. Is it possible to go further? An effort must be made because we all face so many obstacles to our ambitions, and not every obstacle can be the concern of health workers. The stage that has been reached does not go far enough in explaining the nature of health. We need to probe deeper still. The fact that I would like my car sprayed a different colour but cannot afford it because I have not sold enough copies of this book is an obstacle to me, but even I cannot argue that this obstacle should be the direct concern of health workers.

We have discovered from the various theories of health discussed so far that health is not only to do with the physical condition of people. Health is not merely the antithesis of illness and disease. Health is not the sole concern of medicine. Health is not an absolute. It is not something that can be defined precisely. Neither is it something which can be fully described in universal or objective terms—people disagree about the nature of health and have every right to do so. Their opinions are important. It is not the case that only one view out of them all is correct, and that all the others are wrong.

From all this it follows that health is not an ideal to which all people can aspire equally. This may have come as a shock when this point was made in the previous chapter. It sounds divisive and inegalitarian. In fact it is realistic and need be neither divisive nor inegalitarian. It is an inescapable fact that people are naturally unequal. They have different potentials to achieve dependent upon their natural physical and mental capabilities. Although all human beings should be respected equally as human beings, we cannot all be Olympic athletes, nor can we all be prize-winning novelists— some of us just do not have it in us. Different people—the forward child, the terminal patient, the pregnant mother, the inadequately housed—need different conditions to enable them to fulfil their biological and chosen potentials.

What More is Needed in Order to Offer an Adequate Theory of Health?

A comprehensive and useful theory of health needs to take account of the discussion of the previous chapters. It should try to avoid the pitfalls encountered by other theories. A full theory of health also needs to be able to do the following specific tasks:

1. The theory must propose a limit to the legitimate meanings of health, and it must do so as clearly as possible. The theory must be able to acknowledge that there is a great width to the possible uses of the word health, but it must also be able to explain that work for health is not totally comprehensive. Not all aspects of human life are to do with work for health. The World Health Organization makes this mistake with its theory that health is an ideal state of complete physical,

social, and mental wellbeing, which must give all conceivable professions a stake in work for health. Equally it can mean that work for health can impinge on all aspects of people's lives. In a sense this may be true, but we must heed Illich's warning that the medical establishment acts to control too much of our lives. We should not allow health workers to take over this mantle.

2. The theory must recognize that people can disagree about the nature of health and yet all be partially correct. The theory needs to recognize that the conflicts between other theories and approaches cannot be resolved simply by saying that theory X is wrong, theory Y is wrong, theory Z is correct, and so on. The issue is not as simple as this.

   The theory must be able to throw calm on these troubled waters. It must be able to put the overt conflicts into perspective. It must, given that all the theories discussed have some worth, be able to arbitrate between disputes that indicate common ground. The theory must be able to show that although there are real disagreements there need not inevitably be head-on collisions. For instance, the theory must be able to show that it need not necessarily be the case that medical theories of health must confront theories which hold that health is essentially the ability to adapt to all that life throws up. It must show that it is not in every case a matter of the theory that health is a normal functioning in society being directly opposed to the idea that health is strength. Although these theories are set against each other at some levels, the theory must make it clear that the conflicts are not as deep as the agreements about the fundamental goals.

3. The theory needs to be useful. There is little point, other than for intrinsic interest, in abstract debate for its own sake. The theory must be applicable by policy makers, administrators, health educators, medics, nurses, teachers, and neighbours. In fact the theory must be applicable by all individuals on their own behalf, and on the behalf of others in the community.

4. Because it is a mistake to think of health as an absolute, the theory must be able to articulate the idea that there can be *degrees of health*. Issues in health do not boil down to a choice of either/or—either Dennis is healthy or he is not. Without this deeper understanding the case of real Dennis's will forever remain in black and white dispute, with the possible consequence that the help they are given, or can give themselves, will not be clear or will be too restricted.

5. The theory must permit some sort of measurement of health. In order to judge the effectiveness of work for health it must be possible to evaluate people's health, even when health is thought of in the fullest, holistic sense. Without this it will be impossible to come to shared conclusions about the success or failure of work for health.

6. The theory must not appear to be unrealistic. It should not be out of step with current usage. The theory should aim to change not by confronting people, not by saying 'you have been wrong all these years', but by enriching personal concepts of health, by providing people with developed ideas which make sense of work they are doing already. New theories must filter gently into consciousness in order to be taken seriously, in order, in the end, to achieve the goal of changing people's lives for the better. It is a mistake, in more than one sense, to conflict too starkly with accepted use. It must still remain correct to write such slogans as 'Cigarettes can seriously damage your health'. It must still be correct to say 'I have good

health' and mean only that one is in good physical condition. This is a proper comment about health, but it speaks about health in a limited way. Such talk does not invoke the fullest sense of health.

7. The theory must acknowledge the enormous range of factors that can affect the lives of people. The theory must be able to accommodate the width of the fullest sense of health. It must be able to give convincing reasons why health is not simply the antithesis of illness and disease.

This is a very tall order. The theory given in this chapter meets this order. To help make this clear it is worth considering an idea that Socrates put forward, and worth studying a diagram which tries to put words into pictures.

Socrates' Thoughts on Roundness

As we saw earlier with the example of 'justice', Socrates was intrigued by 'what is' questions. He knew that nothing is as simple as it first appears, and that the task of defining does not escape this maxim. Socrates did not attempt to define 'health', as far as we know, but what he did try to do in his inquiries into the meaning of other words is enlightening. For instance, Socrates tried to define 'roundness'. He asked, what does 'being round' mean?

We describe many objects as 'round' even though they are not exactly the same. What are the limits beyond which we would not wish to describe objects as round? Socrates' proposals about this are complicated and involve what is known as The Theory of Forms. Socrates thought that somewhere there exists a perfect and unchanging example of roundness—a standard against which all actual examples of roundness in the real world can only be imperfect copies. All actual examples imitate the perfect form to a recognizable degree. This aspect of Socrates' argument is not important here. It is not helpful, and too similar to the faulty World Health Organization definition, to suggest that there is a perfect essence of health existing eternally somewhere, whilst all actual instances of health in this world are imitations of this perfection.

The reason for introducing one of Socrates' central ideas—albeit in a very oversimplified way—is to point out that *to provide a satisfactory account of something it is not necessary to provide a precise definition. The essential thing to do is to delimit— to show limits beyond which the account becomes unsatisfactory.* Consider the example of 'roundness'. Apples, oranges, rubber balls, cricket balls, and planets are all recognizably round, but we would certainly wish to quibble about other points about these objects which are finer. At the other extreme tables and squares and trees are not round—the limit has clearly been exceeded with these examples. This limit will always be fuzzy at the edges in the real world. For instance, is a plum round? Is an apple with a bite taken out of it round? In practice there will always be uncertainty in some areas.

Within the limit all need not be harmonious. Within the limit there will remain room for conflict and difference. The functions of apples and balls and planets are different. So too are their colours and sizes and textures. But they all share the common feature of roundness.

This topic has been introduced as a device to make it a little easier to understand the point of saying that there is a limit to the sense of health, which can be displayed fairly clearly, and also that within this limit there can be real differences which cannot be, and do not have to be, resolved.

Socrates' idea about the limits to the meaning of 'roundness' can be illustrated in this way:

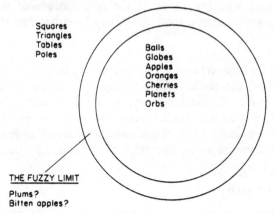

Health is Foundations for Achievement

Work for health is essentially *enabling*. It is a question of providing the appropriate foundations to enable the achievement of personal and group potentials. Health in its different degrees is created by removing obstacles and by providing the basic means by which biological and chosen goals can be achieved.

A person's optimum state of health is equivalent to the state of the set of conditions which fulfil or enable a person to work to fulfil his or her realistic chosen and biological potentials. Some of these conditions are of the highest importance for all people. Others are variable dependent upon individual abilities and circumstances.

The actual degree of health that a person has at a particular time depends upon the degree to which these conditions are realized in practice.

Central Conditions

Some of the foundations which make up health are of the highest importance for all people. These are:

1. The basic needs of food, drink, shelter, warmth, and purpose in life.
2. Access to the widest possible information about all factors which have an influence on a person's life.
3. The skill and confidence to assimilate this information. In most societies literacy and numeracy are needed in older children and adults. People need to be able to understand how the information applies to them, and to be able to make reasoned decisions about what action to take in the light of their information.
4. The recognition that an individual is never totally isolated from other people and the external world. People are complex wholes who cannot be fully understood separated from the influence of their environment, which is itself a whole of which they are a part. People are not like marbles packed in boxes, where they are

a community only because of their forced proximity. People are part of their whole surroundings, like cells in a single body (I thank Dr Michael Wilson for these metaphors). This fact compels the recognition that a person should not strive to fulfil personal potentials which will undermine the basic foundations for achievement of other people. In short, an essential condition for health in human beings who are aware of the implications of their actions is that they have an awareness of a basic duty they have because they are people in a community.

Other foundations for achievement are bound to vary between individuals dependent upon which potentials can realistically be achieved. For instance, a diseased person, a person in a damp and dilapidated house, a person in prison, a fit young athlete, a terminal patient, and an expectant mother all need the central conditions which constitute part of their healths, but in addition they require other specific foundations in order to enable them to make the most of their present lives.

Influences on health

As a small supplement to the vast literature on the extent of the range of factors which can cause disease and illness, research carried out at Wolverhampton Polytechnic has been most revealing. A project was devised to inquire into the anticipated different ways in which different groups of health care professionals think of health. The first stage of the project was to concentrate on the concepts of nurses, and on how these might change during their training. Trainee nurses, qualified nurses, nurse tutors, health visitors, and district nurses were all asked what they think health is. Not unexpectedly the majority of the responses were vague. The World Health Organization's definition was sometimes cited, although it was usually described as 'not right'. If pressed many of the interviewees put forward positions which soon became contradictory.

A different line of attack was tried. The subjects were asked to 'List as many factors as you can which have a bearing on the health of people'. Some of the responses were surprisingly diverse. They included such factors as finance, food/diet, housing/warmth, electricity and gas boards (!), well-woman clinics, environment, family planning associations, smoking, transport, occupations, street lighting, culture, membership of ethnic groups, family pets, the National Health Service, private hospital care, sanitation, sewage, climate, safety factors—home accidents and factory accidents, restaurants, dairies, butchers, sexual relationships, jogging, lack of exercise, sedentary jobs, general practitioners, clothing, anxiety, stress, family pressures, education, unemployment, shopping areas (!), heredity, political decisions, social class, intelligence, crop spraying, other pollution, age, sex, religion, greed, fear, chiropody, government policy, prophylaxis, and the media.

It is clearly much easier to say what affects health than to say what health is. What the research confirmed is that practising health workers think about health in a way that is wider than disease cure and prevention. All these factors are legitimate influences on health according to the theory that health is foundations for achievement. The most commonly identified, and the most important, *influences on health* are those shown in the diagram.

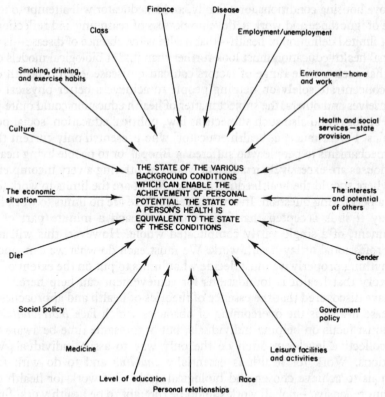

Finance   Disease
Class
Employment/unemployment
Smoking, drinking,
and exercise habits
Environment—home
and work
Culture
Health and social
services—state
provision
THE STATE OF THE VARIOUS
BACKGROUND CONDITIONS
WHICH CAN ENABLE THE
The economic   ACHIEVEMENT OF PERSONAL   The interests
situation   POTENTIAL. THE STATE OF   and potential
A PERSON'S HEALTH IS   of others
EQUIVALENT TO THE STATE
OF THESE CONDITIONS
Diet   Gender
Social policy   Government
policy
Medicine   Leisure facilities
and activities
Level of education   Race
Personal relationships

There are two main ways in which such influences can affect health (i.e. affect the strength of personal foundations):

1. The influences (if they are bad) can create obstacles in their own right. For example, lack of general education, having a black skin, experiencing poor living conditions, or having trouble in forming personal relationships, can severely limit the possibility of a person achieving more than a few of his or her chosen and positive biological potentials.
2. Such influences can create further obstacles of a kind more traditionally associated with health troubles. For example, it is now well known that a person's class and lifestyle can affect the probability of him becoming ill and diseased, that the type of work a person does can make it more or less likely that she will suffer from injury or stress, that smoking can cause disease, and that the permitting of advertising and sports sponsorship by the tobacco companies persuades people to smoke, that poor personal relationships can cause depression and stress, and that lack of education about the way in which the body works can lead to injury.

All legitimate approaches to the creation of health—whether these are overtly political, medical, pastoral, or initiated by health visitors and social workers, for instance—attempt to remove obstacles to the achievement of human potential. These obstacles can be biological, educational, environmental, psychological, political, social, institutional, and so on. A surgeon will remove a tumour, a health visitor will attempt to improve housing conditions for a family, and an educator will attempt to remove the obstacle of ignorance and work to develop powers of reasoning and reflection. Even if the most limited definition of health—that health is the absence of disease—is preferred, traditional health education must look further than just at biological models of disease. Given that such a wide range of factors can cause disease, even if health education was to concentrate solely on helping people to achieve a better physical condition for themselves and others, the subject matter of health education could quite justifiably include biology, and also such subjects as law, political education, social policy, and economics. For instance, a 'health educator' who presented only current theories of cancer mechanisms to people who suffered at Bhopal, or to people living near Seascale whose houses are excessively irradiated, would be offering a very incomplete service.

But where should the health educator stop? What are the limits to work for health? This is a perplexing question. In one real sense there are no limits to work for health, especially if it is accepted that individuals are each a minute part of the total environment, of a single vastly complicated whole. However, this will not do for either professional or lay health work. We must each do what we can, and in order to do anything properly we must decide what limits to put on the extent of our tasks. The theory that health is foundations for achievement can help here.

We have discovered that the essence of theories of health and approaches designed to increase health is the overcoming of obstacles which face *individuals*. Work for health must focus on helping individuals, but at the same time be aware that work at the collective level can often be the only way to assist individuals with their foundations. Work for health is essentially *enabling* and to do with facilitating individuals to achieve chosen and biological goals. But work for health cannot be fully comprehensive—not all work should be thought to be health work. Such a state of affairs is not possible, nor is it desirable to have professional interference in the name of health covering all aspects of individual's lives. *Once suitable background conditions have been created, the achievement of the particular potentials that have been chosen is up to the individual and not the concern of health workers, although permanent maintenance work will often need to be carried out on the foundations.*

The analogy of work for health is very close to the work needed to lay the foundations of a building. *Obstacles such as poor drainage, subsidence, awkward outcrops of rock (analogy: disease, illness, poor housing, discrimination, unemployment) have to be eliminated or overcome in some other way. Then firm foundations and reinforcements have to be added (analogy: good general education, confidence in thinking things through personally rather than relying on what one has been told, good opportunities for self-development). But, unlike the case of building construction, work for health should stop here.* What a person makes of the foundations he has is up to that person, as long as he possesses at least the bones of the central conditions. Given this then an individual must be allowed to become the architect of her own destiny.

The Limits to Health Work

For practical purposes there have to be some limits to work for health. Health workers must be able to decide on priorities, and to focus on specific targets of primary concern for them. The limit to work for health is that it must be work on the foundations or set of conditions necessary for the achievement of some biological and chosen potentials, and also to enable people to develop themselves—to work towards the achievement of other biological and chosen potentials. These potentials must include both body building and intellect building, because people have mental life as well as physical existence.

At this point we can recall Socrates' thoughts on roundness. He believed that it is possible to state the limits of the meaning of this word. However, even in this case the limits are fuzzy. With the case of health the limits are even more fuzzy, but certain workable limits can and must be given.

It is the set of basic conditions which must be of primary concern for health workers, although they must always be aware that, in particular cases, obstacles can be created by a wide range of unexpected factors. The world is an interconnected whole: nothing is finally clear-cut, but the clearest limit possible has to be drawn. *The key is that work for health is work on building a solid stage, and keeping that stage in good condition. The roles that people perform, and how they choose to perform these roles upon that stage is up to the individuals provided that the platform is sound.* For instance, health workers should not interfere once autonomy has been achieved by an individual. It is not the job of work for health to *help* in the achievement of a great many potentials that people may choose, or even to prevent the achievement of chosen potentials even if their achievement will undermine some personal foundations of the individual concerned. In this case choice is paramount.

The **central conditions** given above are the primary targets in work for health.

The limits to the legitimate meanings of health are intimately connected to the limits to health work. The analogue between 'roundness' and 'health' is not perfect. There is more fuzziness to the limits to health work than there is to the limits to the meaning and use of the word 'roundness' for the following reason.

Although it is possible to state the central foundations reasonably clearly, the needs of particular individuals in particular circumstances can be so diverse that work on laying exceptional foundations may have to be done. For instance, it is not normally the job of a health worker to provide books on specialist subjects for people, although health workers should ensure that people understand where they can obtain them for themselves. However, if the person they are trying to help is a prisoner and the prison cannot supply these books, then it is quite legitimate for a health worker, as part of her profession, to provide these books in order to enable the prisoner to begin personal work to develop himself.

What this shows is that on occasions elements which normally lie outside the limits of work for health may enter them briefly. For instance, spending the final hours with a dying person in order to enable that person to achieve better the little potential that is left to them. This is not part of the normal scope of work for health. The normal area of concern is to do with building and maintaining the basic foundations for individual self-development, but a substantial part of a health worker's normal role is vigilance. She must observe and take note of the occasions when tasks which are normally outside the limits of work for health enter these limits temporarily.

What are the analogues of Socrates' squares?

What aspects of life are *not* normally or *not* ever the concerns and targets of work for health?

1. Specific training in specialist subjects. Work for health does not normally involve training people on building and construction courses, or engineering courses, or in foreign languages, or in non-basic maths, for instance.
2. Unproblematic everyday normal activities. For instance, shopping, socializing, and relaxing should not normally concern health workers. A person who is living as a fulfilled member of a society should be left alone by health workers.
3. Personal choosing when a person has the central conditions is never to do with health workers.
4. Health workers should never resort to indoctrination. Such tactics might be appealing on the ground that they are most effective, but indoctrination must be avoided because the long-term effect of its continued use is the undermining of some of the essential conditions which make up individual health.
5. Health workers should never restrict the information available to individuals, even when diverse information conflicts and is contradictory. People should be allowed to arrive at their own conclusions.
6. Health workers should attempt to limit personal choices and potentials only when their fulfilment will undermine the basic foundations of other individuals.
7. Work for health should never encourage or promote activities which will undermine the central and other important foundations of the individual concerned, or which will undermine the foundations of others. For instance, work for health should not encourage disease creating activities, activities which create stress, or activities which are unfulfilling. Work for health can never advocate the dismantling of foundations, but there is an important distinction to be made here. In cases where people do things which undermine important foundations of other people, it may often be possible to intervene directly. For instance, if an individual owns a factory which is seriously polluting a neighbourhood, thus undermining many people's biological foundations, then it may be possible and correct to instigate legal action against the factory owner. However, if an individual who is well aware of the implications of what he is doing to himself chooses to adopt a way of life which undermines some of his important foundations for achievement, then health workers have less power. They may continue to present information about the consequences of this activity, and they may suggest alternatives, but they can do no more than this, and should stop even this work if requested.

According to the theory that health is equivalent to the state of the set of foundations necessary for personal achievement, the task of all health workers must be to provide as strong a set of foundations as possible, but only some are central and needed by all. Great care must be taken to ensure that the other foundations laid are *appropriate*. They must be appropriate to the chosen potentials that a particular person is trying to achieve.

Health workers should constantly reflect on what it is that they are doing when they attempt to promote health. They must ask whether a particular person actually wants what it is that the health worker is trying to give him. Perhaps the 'client' smokes thirty cigarettes per day, drinks about five pints of lager each evening, and eats rich fried food habitually. A question that must be asked is whether it is the 'client's' priority to stop smoking, to moderate his drinking, and to cut down on his carbohydrate—or is he happy doing these things? Will things be worse for him if he does cut down? Are there more pressing obstacles in the way of him achieving a chosen potential? Does he want to move to another area? Does he want a garden? Does he not want a garden? Does he want a different house? Does he need a challenge? Does he need some form of intellectual stimulation? What is the preference of the individual? What is the point of lengthy counselling on the dangers of smoking when the person wants to change his life in some other way, enjoys smoking and is prepared to accept the risks?

If this point is accepted then health workers have accepted that *a person can actively choose to undermine some of his or her foundations for achievement*—in the above case the person is clearly in some danger of impeding his biological potential, and thus his potential to do such things as take part in energetic leisure pursuits. Must health workers accept this conclusion?

They must as long as the person understands clearly what he is doing, but this does not mean that they must stop spreading the ideas in which they believe. Or that they must cease action at a collective level aimed at curbing cigarette and alcohol advertising, production, and consumption. Or that they must give up trying to

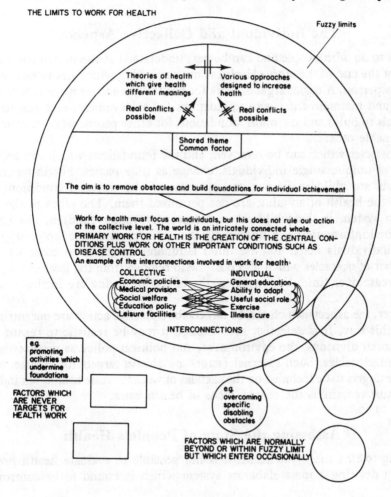

THE LIMITS TO WORK FOR HEALTH

Fuzzy limits

Theories of health which give health different meanings

Various approaches designed to increase health

Real conflicts possible

Real conflicts possible

Shared theme Common factor

The aim is to remove obstacles and build foundations for individual achievement

Work for health must focus on individuals, but this does not rule out action at the collective level. The world is an intricately connected whole. PRIMARY WORK FOR HEALTH IS THE CREATION OF THE CENTRAL CONDITIONS PLUS WORK ON OTHER IMPORTANT CONDITIONS SUCH AS DISEASE CONTROL

An example of the interconnections involved in work for health:

COLLECTIVE
Economic policies
Medical provision
Social welfare
Education policy
Leisure facilities

INDIVIDUAL
General education
Ability to adapt
Useful social role
Exercise
Illness cure

INTERCONNECTIONS

e.g. promoting activities which undermine foundations

FACTORS WHICH ARE NEVER TARGETS FOR HEALTH WORK

e.g. overcoming specific disabling obstacles

FACTORS WHICH ARE NORMALLY BEYOND OR WITHIN FUZZY LIMIT BUT WHICH ENTER OCCASIONALLY bring about changes in the thinking and lifestyles of groups, communities, and societies.

Although the fullest individual health is achieved when—given certain restrictions imposed by the real world, such as personal circumstances, laws, the interests of other people, social norms, and structure—a person is unimpeded in the pursuit of his or her *chosen potentials* as well as in the achievement of his or her *biological potentials*, choice must be paramount. This is so with the proviso that this choice is based on personal reflection and consideration of the consequences. People are more than biological units.

Further differences arise in two respects:

1. It is a fact that not all chosen or biological potentials can be achieved by individuals because, as is illustrated by the above example, not all potentials are compatible.
2. The line which divides the areas in which health workers are justified in intervening directly, and those where they can only advise, is not sharp. In practice tough questions about how much an individual's actions are affecting other people for the worse frequently have to be faced.

The Individual and Collective Aspects

Health is to do with people and can be best understood at the individual level, but this is not the end of the story. Health is not something which has to be constantly given to a person. A basic target of work for health is to encourage people to be able to build and maintain their own foundations for achievement, and also to enable individuals to build and maintain foundations for other people who, in turn will be able to enable others.

The obstacles which can be removed, and the foundations which can be laid, in the case of unique single individuals, change as time passes. For instance, when individuals are children in our society some of the essential conditions which make up the health of an adult are not permitted them. The ethos of the British education system is that children, and especially young children, can be given only limited information and limited choices. This practice is adopted in order to prepare individuals better for the fuller autonomy which is to come later. Also the number of obstacles which it is possible to remove from the lives of individuals may decrease over time. For instance, the effects of ageing are intrinsic personal features.

However, the aspects which can be targets for collective action are not intrinsically fixed in this way. It is defeatist, even though it may be realistic to regard factors such as social divisions, the environment, and political policy as necessarily being permanent obstacles. Such external factors are always targets for change, and are legitimate targets to be included on the agendas of work to create health, but individual people must remain as the central focus of health work.

Assessing the State of People's Health

According to this theory of health it is not possible to evaluate health precisely, except by devising a most elaborate system which is bound to be controversial.

However, it is possible, and very useful for practitioners, to have some idea about how to distinguish between different levels of health. If it is true that the level of a person's health is directly related to the strength of the foundations which have been laid, then it is possible to have a loose idea of that person's health. A person's health will be dependent on the amount and range of obstacles which have been eliminated and overcome, and on the quality and quantity of the background conditions that have been provided. In this sense health is equivalent to the amount of freedom of choice and action that a person has.

It is not the purpose of this book to develop a full system by which health can be quantified. It is possible to imagine such a system. For instance, different obstacles to achievement could be given different negative values dependent on how serious a liability each is, and different enabling conditions could be given different positive values dependent upon how enhancing each is. For example, diseases could be measured on such a system dependent upon such factors as how disabling they are, how long they persist, and how life-threatening they are. Other liabilities which might possibly be roughly quantified are poor housing, lack of knowledge, and illiteracy, for instance. Such negative weightings could be counter-balanced by the positive values of the features in people's foundations for achievement which will enhance lives.

This sort of system of measurement would be unwieldy and contentious. No objective standards could be proposed without persisting dispute, but if people are willing to accept a fairly high level of imprecision such a system could provide a rough guide to a person's state of health, along a continuum which takes account of a host of factors. Crudely:

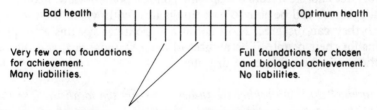

The *degrees of health* in between make it possible to talk
of a person having fair or even good health in the presence
of liabilities such as disease, injury and illness

It is a serious mistake to assume that such a system is the same as that which has been proposed to measure a person's quality of life in certain cases where resources for medical treatment are in short supply. That system assumes that positive potentials are as fixed as the negative personal circumstances. This is an inexcusable pessimism which this theory of health is designed to combat. Work for health is work to enable. A permanent central question is 'how can we provide more enabling conditions for this individual?'

The idea that there can be degrees of health can be illuminating. This will be seen when it is loosely applied to the case studies we met earlier.

What is wrong with this theory?

There are a number of objections that can be made to this theory. Certainly there will be more than are listed below. These objections can be answered, at least in part.

1. *The theory is just one person's idea of health. We have been told that health cannot be defined, and that there can be no universally acceptable theories of health. This theory is just as good, and just as bad, as any of the others.*

Response There are no totally objective standards against which to measure the worth of theories, but there are other standards. This theory shows where other theories of health are inadequate and insufficiently thought through; it argues that certain areas should be primary targets for health workers, and it provides a crude way of assessing health and is thus a gauge for practical work. It is more specific than other theories. As a result it will be far easier to show where it slips up, and to suggest improvements. In all these things the theory that health is foundations for achievement is an advance on previous theories of health.

2. *The theory is an argument for political and social change which uses health as a convenient and emotive platform. It is just one more instance of band-wagon jumping.*

Response The theory is an argument for social change. It can apply to any society. Some societies need changing more than others.
   The idea of health is focused on because so many people work in the name of health, and so much is written about health, without those who do the work and the writing being fully clear about what they are doing or what they mean. The theory does not try to use health as an emotive platform. The genesis of this inquiry was a genuine compulsion to clarify the meaning of health.
   The theory does not stem from one specific political point of view. People of different political allegiances will be able to find things in it with which they can agree, and with which they can disagree. Most social and political systems attempt to create foundations for their people. The natures of these foundations, and the method of their creation, are the subjects of disputes.

3. *The thinking which lies behind the theory is simply too idealistic. The theory tries to point the way to a utopia.*

Response In a sense this is true, but people should have visions. We need ideals, so long as we realise that this is what they are.
   For everyone to have the fullest degree of health possible for them as unique individuals there would have to be tremendous social, political and economic upheavals. Real work for health does not strive directly for such huge goals. Since work for health focuses on the individual, and recognizes that individuals can never be divorced from their wider environments, it is possible to increase health by small degrees. The hope is that these small steps multiply and progress accelerates.
   It has been argued by Marxist thinkers and others that there is a contradiction here. It is said that by just trying to help people in small ways health workers 'patch up' the existing social system—they reinforce it by helping people to operate again in the very system which created their ill-health. This objection would be true if health workers do not at the same time try either to improve existing systems or to change them altogether. Which is better: to leave people to suffer when you have the power to improve their lives in some ways, in the hope that all this suffering

will somehow bring about change; or help people cope within the situation that exists, and also promote the idea as widely as possible that the existing system could be altered? Care at a personal level rarely reinforces a system. This sort of care simply is not scrutinized by 'the system'.

It is also a real possibility that by working to provide the *central conditions* universally, other wider changes will occur as a result.

4.   *The theory is not fully worked out.*

Response   This is true. It is developed further in Chapter Seven. Theories take time to grow. They need to be put to work and criticized.

Chapter Six
The Idea of Human Potential

The idea of human potential requires clarification. 'Potential' is one of the notorious 'keywords' which, if care is not taken, can generate a verbal smokescreen, convenient or otherwise.

The theory of health offered in this book argues that *a person's health is equivalent to the state of the set of conditions which fulfil or enable a person to work to fulfil his or her realistic chosen and biological potentials*. Roughly this means that if a person has a broad and sound set of conditions which fulfil or enable him to achieve certain potentials, then his health is good. If the set of fulfilling or enabling conditions is small and the conditions weak, then his health is poor. This theory is an advance on other theories. It strikes a hopeful chord, but it poses further questions which cannot be avoided.

The two main questions are: *What is meant by 'realistic'?* and *What is meant by 'potential'?*

1. What is Meant by the Term 'Realistic' in this Theory?

It seems to read rather like a 'get-out clause', but it is not meant in this way. It could be taken to be an acceptance of fatalism. For instance, it could be taken to signify that a working-class child from a 'broken home' should accept that the limit on the positive and fulfilling goals he can achieve in his life is low, that he has been given his lot and he should be realistic about it. If this meaning were to be intended then the theory would be sadly pessimistic, but this meaning is not intended.

The word 'realistic' is included in the definition put forward to make it clear that the theory does not aspire to the World Health Organization's goal of complete physical, mental and social wellbeing. Such a utopia cannot be achieved in this world. It is intended to warn against wishful thinking and working towards impossible chosen goals, but it is intended mainly to refer to biological potentials. In order to improve physically a person must be realistic about her present condition, and about the speed and direction of change that is possible. Biological potentials inevitably change as diseases and illnesses are suffered, and as people age.

To sum up: the idea of realism is included in order to make the point that in order to achieve the various potentials that an individual has, a start has to be made from the state he has *now*. This applies to the biological and chosen potentials of individuals, but the idea of realism is not included to foster fatalistic attitudes to life. Although part of the present condition of any individual rests on many elements that are intrinsic to that individual, external circumstances are not fixed in the same way. Class divisions and other injustices can be changed.

2.   What is Meant by 'Potential'?

Assumptions are made in any theory. It is best to be as clear as possible about those that the theorist is clear about.

Assumptions

1. This assumption continues the anti-fatalism theme. A person is not merely living out a pre-determined destiny which he is powerless to alter. Except in extreme instances of illness or external control (such as solitary confinement without external stimulus), people possess an indefinite number of potentials depending upon what they do, and what happens to them. We all have physical and intellectual potential until we die. Although what has already become actual may increasingly affect that which is still potential, what has happened to our bodies will limit us in a physical sense, and what has happened to our minds will limit us intellectually, there will always remain the potential to achieve a range of possibilities.

    This is true even of terminal patients in hospital, even until the time they finally lapse into unconsciousness. Not only do such people have choices about which potentials to achieve for themselves, they also have the potential to influence other people such as their friends, families, and carers, in different ways. A dying person might be depressed and self-pitying. She might be pathetic. Or she might inspire, set the example she would wish to have set for her, give love and be loved. She might talk to people in a way she has never done before, and she might see them, and they see her, in a different light.

    Throughout a human life a person has a host of latent potentials, which in general will decrease with time. Not all of these potentials can be achieved. Much depends upon circumstances. Some doors open, stay ajar for a while, and then close permanently. Sportsmen often choose to specialize, so shutting many doors as they go through one. Sometimes surprising doors open. For instance, many life prisoners have or are taking university degrees, thus fulfilling a potential that almost certainly would never have been realized in normal circumstances.
2. This theory of health takes an optimistic view of life. It assumes that people can change themselves and their environments for the better. It assumes that they will want to, and that they will wish the improved conditions they enjoy to be enjoyed by others. It assumes that people do not, and certainly do not have to, think of their potentials only in a selfish way.

Can people's potentials be assessed?

There are sayings to the effect that '. . . give me a boy at seven and I'll show you the man . . .', and '. . . I always knew that he'd turn out to be a bad 'un . . .'. There is something in such dictums. People do have certain attributes and characteristics which remain with them throughout life.

There are some tests which can be carried out in order to assess potential. For instance, doctors can judge the adult height of a child fairly accurately. People have genetic potentials which determine their biological development. IQ tests can be done to determine the level of ability of parts of people's intellects, but *the potential of a person is not the same as the potential of an engine*—where the maximum possible efficiency can be stated. There is, thankfully, a high degree of uncertainty about which potentials people will achieve. Children confidently predicted by consensus to be potential 'bad 'uns' can turn out to be caring, clergymen, philosophers, policemen, burglars, or whatever the opposite of '. . . being a bad 'un . . .' is. The child of seven may have fixed characteristics which can be identified, but a study of the seven-year-old will not show what will happen to the man, or how he will deal with external events in his 'characteristic way'.

Problem: not all potentials are good

People are potentially evil, senile, diseased, dead, and stupid. We have the potential to be jealous, malicious, and selfish. We can and do injure, abuse, and impede other people. The problem is that if work for health is work to remove various obstacles to the achievement of human potentials, then why should health workers not remove obstacles which prevent the achievement of the kinds of potentials which are normally regarded to be bad?

How can positive and negative potentials be distinguished?

No absolute distinction can be made. There are occasions when some 'bad potentials' ought to be achieved, and questions of value are always disputed. However, it is possible to put forward a working distinction.

Work for health is concerned with enabling fulfilling achievements. It aims for the achievement of normative or positive potentials. Medicine is an example of a means which is employed to help people achieve norms. For instance, it is accepted that 'normal bodies' and 'normal children' will develop in certain predictable ways, such is their normative potential. If they are developing abnormally then steps might be taken to attempt to bring them nearer to a normal state—unless they are regarded as exceptional or prodigies!

Ideas about 'positive potentials' will vary, but what is common to the notion of positive potential is that individuals will seek to achieve a range of states which they believe will *enhance* their lives in a variety of ways. For instance, people might aim to improve physically—by exercising, by dieting, by cosmetic surgery, by other surgery—or intellectually—by reading and taking courses of education—or socially, or emotionally. Not all people will see these goals as positive, but they will recognize personally enhancing potentials and set about fulfilling them.

The idea of 'positive potential' can be contrasted with the idea of *liability*. Liabilities are the sorts of problem which act against the achievement of positive or normative potential. For instance, disease is a liability which, if circumstances had been different need not have occurred. Ignorance is a liability which, if not overcome, can prevent the achievement of all sorts of positive potential. Negative potentials are liabilities.

It is possible to strip this distinction of at least some of its ambiguity. Work for health is work which aims to enable and to enhance by providing foundations for the achievement of potentials. It is opposed to liabilities because they are debilitating. The distinction hinges on the difference between the ideas of *enhancing* and *debilitating*.

Work for health will be concerned with encouraging normative and positive potentials because these potentials have the effect of opening up possibilities for achieving more potentials, whereas negative potentials reduce the number of possible potentials. This reduction is often severe.

Examples of positive potential are higher standards of reasoning ability, greater assimilation of knowledge, and an increased level of ability to develop oneself autonomously. Examples of negative potential are the potential to commit suicide, the potential to be diseased, and the potential to despair.

The role of health workers in the achievement of potentials

The potentials which concern health workers are not the negative, debilitating ones. Health workers are concerned to enable, to widen and to increase the possibilities for achievement. Health workers are not in the business of laying foundations for potentials which *in themselves* can be considered to be obstacles. Health workers should aim to provide the central and other relevant important conditions. They should aim to counter ignorance, lack of reasoning ability, selfishness, disease, illness, and injury.

Health workers naturally do not wish the people they have enabled then to undermine their own foundations, or to undermine the foundations for achievement of others, but health workers must remember that choice is a central condition, and that their work stops at work on the foundations. Health workers do not look over the shoulder of a person doing a physics examination, attending a job interview, signing a contract for a house, or sealing a business deal. Individual liberty must be respected. Health workers have no right or duty—other than the legal duties of all citizens in some cases—to prevent a person autonomously choosing a potential with which the health worker disagrees, or which the health worker knows will undermine the given or self-created foundations of that person. For instance, if a person is fully aware of the implications of what he proposes to do, and he wishes to abuse his body in some way then he must be allowed to do so, although work to show him information which might make him change his mind can continue. Work for health is work to provide the basic foundations for achievement, and then to try to maintain these so that a person always has the widest possible choice about which potentials she wishes to achieve.

Chapter Seven
The Assessment of the Health of Individuals

Two central questions are considered in this chapter. They are: *Which of the case studies is healthy and which unhealthy?* and *How could each case study become more healthy?*

Which of the Case Studies is Healthy and Which Unhealthy?

This question was left unanswered at the end of Chapter One. The result of this initial inquiry was most unsatisfactory. Not one of the hypothetical people discussed was said to be healthy by all the various definers of health. Dennis, Anne, Mr James and Peter were all described as healthy twice and as unhealthy twice. The medic, the social scientist, the idealist, and the humanist could not agree about the states of health of the case studies, which was not surprising since they each have different ideas about the nature of health.

It was decided at the end of Chapter One that the overall inquiry of the book was not sufficiently advanced to allow a more satisfactory assessment of the case studies. More progress has now been made. The theories and definitions of health preferred by the various specialists have now been analysed, and their defects have been revealed. None of these theories has been sufficiently thought through by the respective theorists to be used in an assessment of a person's health. A new theory of health has been put forward. It is complicated and contentious, but it is sufficiently developed to be applied. By using this theory it is possible to reach a considered opinion about the state of health of individuals.

It is a mistake to think that a person's state of health can be measured precisely. There are far too many contestable variables involved, but if work for health is to mean anything it must be possible to have a fair idea of the level of health achieved by individuals, and of the nature of new levels of health at which to aim.

In its broadest form the new theory of health advanced in this book states that *a person's health is equivalent to the state of the set of conditions which fulfil or enable a person to work to fulfil his or her realistic chosen and biological potentials. Some of these conditions are of the highest importance for all people. Others are variable dependent upon individual abilities and circumstances.*

Some of these foundations are central, primary conditions which can greatly enable all human beings. These are basic needs such as food, shelter, and purpose in life; access to a very wide range of information about all the factors which have an influence on a person's life; skill and confidence at reasoning with and about this information; and the recognition that a person has a duty not to harm another person in any respect—that work for health can and should involve all human beings.

Other foundations are important although not necessarily central. To give examples: these important foundations can be created by such means as elimination of disease in a person, by counselling and providing wide information to an expecting mother about the various methods of birth possible; by providing a young tennis player with information about her body and her emotions, and about the histories of similar young women, and by informing her about the various choices she could make; or by helping a person to understand how to move from a poor residence to a better one—again foundations can be created by displaying various possibilities, and by continuing to display these possibilities for as long as is necessary.

Work for health involves removing obstacles to the achievement of these potentials, and building firm foundations where necessary. Once suitable background conditions have been created then the achievement of the particular chosen potentials is up to the individual, and not the concern of health workers, although they are responsible for any maintenance work on these foundations.

The *central conditions* are not all required in order for a person to have any degree of health at all, but without any of these an adult or older child will have only a very low level of health, even if she is not diseased or ill.

The assessment of a person's health is not a black and white issue. It is not the case that either a person is healthy or he is not. People and their circumstances are infinitely variable. People's health must be considered in levels. Health can be assessed in degrees.

The issue is even more complicated than this. It is not as if there is a single graded measure against which all people's health can be assessed. All that it is possible to have is a general idea of the states of the various different sets of conditions, which do not even remain constantly required by a single individual.

As we have seen, health can be thought of as a continuum which takes account of a host of factors:

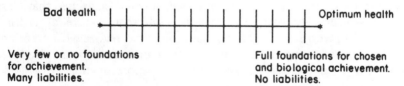

These foundations are not all fixed requirements. The same *idea* can be applied to person A and person B, but they may have different needs.

This degree of vagueness must be recognized. Not to do so is worse than not being able to measure health at all. However, it is now possible to state in general terms, what degree of health a person has. It is also possible to state to what extent one person can have better health, either in general or in some respects, than another.

The new theory of health focuses attention on people's foundations for achievement. An assessment can be made to establish which foundations enable to what degree, to see what obstacles are present, and to discover what liabilities need to be removed.

An Assessment of the States of Health of the Case Studies

Percy

Percy is the ex-office worker who, for the last three years, has been suffering from occasional temporary involuntary delusions where he believes he is, and acts as if he is, another person. During the time he suffers these delusions he cannot interact normally with other people, so he finds it very hard to hold down a job.

Percy has a low level of health. He has not been lucky. His persistent delusions are a major liability. They present a large obstacle in the path of a number of potentials he might have chosen to fulfil. He does not have no health at all. He has several existing foundations for achievement. He has warmth and shelter, he has a lot of information available to him, he understands his problem and he is trying to do something about it. If he found anyone else with a similar problem he would do what he could to help them. The trouble is that, because of this huge obstacle, Percy is unable to build on the foundations he has.

How can Percy's health be improved?   What is needed is the elimination of the impediment. Some way must be found to rid Percy of his curse. If it is found, or if the problem disappears naturally, then Percy will need help with another *central condition*, which we all require anyway. He will need to be helped to recognize a purpose in his life.

If this could be done then Percy's level of health would increase dramatically.

Dennis

Dennis is the lazy, apathetic bank clerk. He is not diseased and does not feel ill. He spends his time at the work he has been doing for the last twenty years, watching his television, or sleeping.

Dennis' case shows that decisions about a person's state of health can often be hotly disputed. If Dennis truly wants to live the way he does then he has all the foundations necessary for the fulfilment of his chosen potential. His biological potential does not seem to be seriously threatened by his lifestyle. It could be argued that Dennis has a high level of health. Alternatively it could be said that his level of health is fairly low. The problem with Dennis may be that he does not realize what other potentials he has, that he needs stimulus and wider information about what else he *could* be doing in order to ensure that he has a greater purpose in life.

How can Dennis's health be improved?   If he does not possess this wider information then he should be shown a range of possibilities that he could choose to do instead of continuing to drift idly. There are countless fulfilling ways in which he could spend his spare time. If he does possess extensive information about choices open to him, and he still prefers to live as he does, then there is nothing further that can or should be done for Dennis at present.

Anne

Anne is the paraplegic journalist. Her body was shattered in a car accident, but she has managed to rebuild her career as a journalist. She has a warm and convenient flat, she has become reconciled to her disability and is now content, and she always tries to encourage other people with their lives and projects.

Anne has a very high level of health even though she is severely handicapped. She has all the *central enabling conditions*, as well as other important foundations, such as her specially designed flat and her assured income, that are appropriate to enable her to achieve her chosen and biological potentials.

How can Anne's health be improved? Anne has a full and appropriate set of enabling conditions at the moment. She has sound foundations for achievement which are enabling her to fulfil her realistic chosen and biological potentials.

It is the idea of realism that is important here. If her handicap could be cured, which is not likely, then she would regain a very important and enabling foundation, but she knows that her injury is permanent. It is now part of her and she knows that she must accept this. If she continued to hope unrealistically, if she fantasized about a return to the way she was, then this wishful thinking would itself become a liability. Her regrets and false hopes would be an obstacle to the achievement of the many positive potentials she still has.

Betty

Betty is the widow with secondary cancer of the brain. She is miserable, frightened, and very worried about the behaviour of her youngest son, but she has great character and is fighting her disease with all the strength that she has.

Although Betty has a serious disease she is not totally unhealthy. She has several degrees of health. She has warmth, shelter, and a purpose in life. She understands what is happening to her body and is well educated in other respects. She also cares deeply about what happens to her son. She has a number of foundations on which to build, and one major liability—her cancer.

How can Betty's health be improved? Clearly Betty's level of health would improve if her cancer was cured, or if she had a remission of the disease. In this case the medical profession has a legitimate and important interest in an individual's state of health. But nothing is ever totally good or totally bad. Even cancer has some benefit. It has brought out a side to Betty—her character and strength—which neither she nor her son realized she had.

The James family

Mr and Mrs James are the couple, both twenty years old, who live in damp conditions without electricity. Mrs James is pregnant and in despair. She has no disease. Mr James also does not have a disease but is on probation and cannot get a job. Their child has a low level of speech for his age, and suffers bronchitis and temper tantrums.

Collectively the family has a poor level of health, and each member of the family, considered individually, has a poor level of health. Many *central* and important foundations for achievement are missing. The family has shelter but no warmth, and little purpose in life. They have very limited access to the information about the factors which are shaping their lives, and they do not know how to assimilate this information, or how to use it for their benefit. They feel isolated and, understandably, are concerned only to improve their own lives, if possible.

How can the health of the James family be improved? Radical action is called for. The family has numerous positive potentials and could be enabled to achieve them.

They need electricity and a warm, dry place to live. They need to be shown how to cope better with their money, their relationships, and with contraception. Above this they need a good general education, not only information about such things as bronchitis and the dangers of Valium. They need to know many things that they do not, including the reasons why their flat was built in the first place, and why Mr James cannot find work. They need to understand more about what is happening to them in order to be able to try to do something about their lives. The child needs special attention with his speech, and Mr and Mrs James need to be shown how to enable the child to fulfil more of his potentials.

Winston

Winston is the young, unemployed black man who has been involved in riots, and who deals in 'soft drugs'. He is in excellent physical condition.

As with Dennis, the state of Winston's health is highly contestable. It could be argued that he is fulfilling a high level of physical potential, and that he has most of the *central conditions* at least in part, and so should be considered to have a fairly high level of health. On the other hand it could be said, legitimately, that Winston has much potential which he cannot fulfil because of the prejudice he suffers because of the colour of his skin.

How can Winston's health be improved?   Winston needs more purpose in life. Many of his potentials cannot be tapped because of the obstacle posed by the prejudice of some police and some employers against black people.

Peter

Peter is the successful businessman who enjoys a very high standard of living according to Western standards. He smokes and drinks quite heavily, and is often frustrated and loses his temper.

Peter is well educated and well housed, and he does care about the welfare of other people. He has all the *central conditions* to a degree, and he also has other important foundations for achievement. He chooses to smoke and drink, knowing the possible unfavourable implications of his habits. He is not diseased.

Consequently he has a high level of health. He has firm foundations on which to build his next chosen potentials, although he may be undermining the foundations of his biological potential through his lifestyle and his stress.

This is not to say that the more money a person has the more health he has, but in a capitalist society people need a certain amount of money in order to fulfil much of their potential. Not enough information has been given about his relationship with his wife for his violence to have a bearing on this assessment.

How can Peter's health be improved?   Once again opinions will vary and be arguable. Value judgements cannot be avoided in health issues.

Conclusion

Any assessment of the health of individuals according to the new theory of health will be controversial, even though in many respects the theory is not new at all.

It is now well known that a person's way of life can influence his chances of becoming diseased and ill. It is only one or two steps further to say that *a person's health is intimately linked with his quality of life.*

The method of assessment based on the new theory of health has advantages over alternatives:

1. It makes concrete a way of thinking positively about health. It goes further than the idea that health is the absence or the opposite of disease.
2. It focuses much fuller attention on the wider aspects to people's lives, rather than concentrating only on conditions and cures recognized by medicine. Attention is focused more widely than just on health at the collective level of existing public health and environmental initiatives. It focuses attention on ways of improving health which are far more comprehensive than those proposed by the existing health service. It also has the welcome by-product of indicating ways of preventing disease and illness.
3. It enables health workers to identify the most significant targets to be changed. Health workers can assess which are the most serious obstacles to remove, and which are the most essential enabling conditions to provide.
4. It throws a bright spotlight on the vast and unnecessary inequalities of opportunity which exist between different people in societies.

Chapter Eight
The Aims of Health
Education and Promotion

Introduction

At present the funding of health education and promotion is being increased. The idea is that prevention of disease, illness and injury is better, and cheaper, than curing them. It is possible to study for a certificate of health education, and to take postgraduate diplomas in health education. The subjects offered under this umbrella include communication skills, social policy, environmental health, social medicine, epidemiology, psychology, sociology, organization studies, and statistics and research design. The aim of these courses is to train professional health educators to educate lay-people about health, and also to show them how to promote it.

As far as the promotion of health in its full sense, in the sense of the new theory of health is concerned, these courses—and the work of many qualified health educators and promoters—are inadequate. Despite the good intentions of those involved present health education and promotion strategies fall short on two main counts:

1. Although the various theories discussed in Chapter Four of this book are known, and it is generally acknowledged that health is a very wide 'concept', the practical effect of health education is still to concentrate on preventing diseases, illness and injuries. Health educators try to inform people about smoking, alcohol, and drug abuse; about 'foot health' and 'dental health'; about safety in the home and at work; and about the benefits and dangers of physical exercise. These topics are important, and there is no reason why these ideas should not be explained and promoted, but they are only a limited part of true health education.
2. The major theme of current health education and promotion is *prevention*. However, since a person's health is inextricably linked to her quality of life, the primary aim of health education and promotion should be to *create*.

In one sense this creation can be seen as prevention. It can be seen as the prevention of ignorance, the prevention of the abuse of human beings by social systems, and the prevention of the waste of innumerable personal potentials and talents. People are complex, unique, profound, and always important, however unfortunate their current circumstances. But people are not always permitted the right foundations on which to build *themselves*. Without these foundations people are shaky, incomplete, and liable to collapse. All work for health must be work to provide these foundations.

Present health education and promotion works to prevent at a level which is not the most fundamental, rather like trying to dam a stream half-way down a mountain instead of at its source. The main aims of health education and promotion must be to provide most of the *central conditions* presented in Chapter Five, particularly conditions 2, 3, and 4.

What is Education?

Although the nature of health has been made more clear in this book, no attempt has yet been made to clarify the nature of education. This will not be done in any detail because, unlike the case of health, there have been philosophical debates about the nature and goals of education since the times of the ancient Greeks. The question is as difficult and complex as 'What is Health?'

Nonetheless it is possible to make a fairly clear distinction between the idea of training and the idea of education.

Training

The idea of training is closest to the idea of indoctrination, which is a process which involves imparting a single set of ideas. Training is proper and necessary in disciplines such as computing and engineering, where correct techniques and formulae must be learnt. The importance of a thorough training in many practical disciplines cannot be overestimated, but it is improper and debilitating where human values, lives, and goals are concerned.

Education

True education is a process which aims to achieve two principal goals:

1. To provide the learner, either directly or indirectly, with all relevant information about a subject area.
2. To instil a childlike curiosity which can disappear all too easily; to encourage a questioning attitude, a confidence to select and to criticize; to promote the sense that the information that is being presented is what we have now—it is not the final word; and to encourage the idea that each of us is part of a continuing inquiry. True education enables a person by cultivating his skill to choose autonomously. Simply to present the information, the theories, and the techniques is mechanics. It is not education but a form of programming.

If both goals are aimed for then—given the inevitable real-world limits to autonomy, such as legal rules and the interests of other human beings—it is possible to educate people to be autonomous. It is possible to educate people to the point where they realize that their opinions, theories and experiences are important not only to themselves but also to other people. It is possible to educate people to the point where they regain their philosophical ability.

There are many problems with this point of view, but this is not the place to discuss them.

Health Education should not Indoctrinate.
It should not be a Propaganda Exercise

There are two main reasons for this.

1. Indoctrination undermines the *central conditions* that people should have the fullest
    possible information about factors which affect their lives, and that they should
    have sufficient ability and range of information to make their own reasoned choices.

A useful means of illustrating this point arrived in the mail recently. It is a 'Heart
Chart' sent out by members of a newly established 'Well-man Centre'. The Centre
is interested in helping people live 'healthier lives in the sense of helping them increase
their physical fitness. The Centre aims to help people to achieve their biological norms.
    The chart is intended to help people avoid heart disease. It displays a 'traffic-light'
warning system. If the green light is achieved then all is well, if the amber light is
indicated then this is a warning to a person to change some factors in his life-style,
and if the red light is achieved then this is a warning to stop some habits altogether.
There are ten factors, such as smoking, drinking, eating fried foods, and exercising,
which can contribute to or help prevent heart disease, according to this chart.
Dependent on a person's habits—perhaps she exercises once a week, has little or
no stress, and so on—points can be allocated. The best score for each of the ten
categories is 0 and the worst 4. If the total score is less than 10 then a person gets
a green light, between 10 and 20 he gets an amber light, and between 20 and 40
a red light.
    The thinking behind the chart is well-meaning but it gives little real information,
and is of little help in making a personal choice. Why should smoking increase heart
disease? What are the statistics? I'm half the size of my brother so should I eat less
fried food than him? We've never had any heart trouble in our family so should I
heed these warnings? These are reasonable questions which ought to be answered
in any serious attempt to educate. The 'Heart Chart' happens to be a particularly
good example of the dangers of not giving sufficient information, and of attempting
propaganda. Without further information a person could genuinely be seriously misled.
A person could smoke eighty cigarettes a day and get thoroughly drunk every night,
score 0 on the other eight factors, achieve a total score of eight and so get a green light!

2. Opinions about even the traditional subjects of health education are divided. There
    is always a degree of uncertainty, and people should be made aware of this.

Professor Michael Oliver, President of the British Cardiac Society, reinforced this
point in August 1985. He rejects a currently favoured idea that low fat diets can
save people from heart attacks. In his opinion public health campaigns to reduce
the death toll caused by heart disease by changing life-styles nationwide is simplistic.
Professor Oliver agrees that smoking is a factor in heart disease, but argues that once
smoking is excluded most people who suffered coronary disease had none of the other
supposed risk factors. The causes of heart disease seem to be diverse, and their analysis
and understanding is complicated and uncertain. All the causes of heart disease may
not be known, and those which affect one person's heart need not necessarily affect

another person's heart. He was quoted as saying, 'Such is the force of the juggernaut that has been set forth by these propagandists that little credence is given to genuine scientific doubts. Much of the zeal has arisen from the enthusiasts allowing themselves to be coerced.

'Many health professionals ignore, and some are ignorant, of alternative approaches to coronary heart disease. We must go on with some forms of health education campaigns, but there are many other things to consider.'

Professor Oliver has a specialist's interest in, and view of, health, but he makes a sound general point. Educating, promoting, or working in other ways for the health of others, and working for an individual's own health, is never a matter of following fixed policies or given rules without thinking. Smoking, eating butter, or drinking alcohol regularly, are not activities which are unequivocally anti-health. For instance, Bill Werbeniuk, who is a snooker player, claims to need fourteen pints of lager beer a day in order to play to the best of his ability, a potential to which he gives higher priority than the physical wellbeing of his liver. Also smoking can ease nervousness and tension, and can help with camaraderie. It may cause lung disease, but all drugs have side-effects.

People must be allowed to exercise choice, and the fullest choice can come only from possession of the fullest relevant information.

The Central Aims of Health Education

These should be:

1. *To ensure that all people have a good standard of general education*

The philosopher Paul Feyerabend has written:

> . . . one thing must be avoided at all costs: the special standards which define special subjects and special professions must not be allowed to permeate *general* education and they must not be made the defining property of a 'well-educated man.' General education should prepare a citizen to *choose between* the standards, or to find his way in a society that contains groups committed to various standards *but it must under no condition bend his mind so that it conforms to the standards of one* particular group. The standards will be *considered*, they will be *discussed*, children will be encouraged to get proficiency in the more important subjects, *but only as one gets proficiency in a game*, that is, without serious commitment and without robbing the mind of its ability to play other games as well. Having been prepared in this way a young person may decide to devote the rest of his life to a particular profession and he may start taking it seriously forthwith. This 'commitment' should be the result of a conscious decision, on the basis of a fairly complete knowledge of alternatives, *and not a foregone conclusion*. (Feyerabend, 1978, pp. 217–218)

The state of an individual that Feyerabend urges is a *central condition* for health. If a person does not have this state to a fair degree then one of her central foundations is weak. This is inevitably a concern for health educators, and it is a great challenge too. If such a state could be achieved universally then we would have a shifting, vivacious, exciting, free society.

To disregard this argument is to be accessory to the sacrifice of a latent genius possessed by all people, and to sacrifice the creative spirit which is present in the 'living statues' which are described by Oliver Sacks, on the altar of conservatism, tradition, mediocrity, and fixed order. To ignore the argument is to deny choice. As such it is the asphyxiation of morality. The key to health is to allow people to develop themselves.

2. To develop people's powers of conceiving, and so to enable them to make the most of the information they have

Why was so much time spent on the discussion of concepts and conceiving earlier? It was done to illustrate a point but also to help focus attention on the often latent ability of *conceiving* (intellectually!) that all people possess. The time was spent to begin to focus attention on the importance of each human being.

John Berger's observation of the depth which all people have

The writer John Berger is concerned about the poverty of the human condition. In his book, *A Fortunate Man* (Berger and Mohr, 1976), he relates some of the experiences of John Sassall, a fictional country doctor—who was created by Berger from observation of real life cases—who meets birth, suffering, and death as part of his daily work. Sassall feels empathy with his patients but, although he is glad to have his own fortunate circumstances, he feels frustrated that only he amongst the community in which he practises possesses the words and education necessary to *articulate his thoughts* and so to protest about the emptiness and powerlessness of the human lives he encounters. It is not that people do not have the potential to be able to live fulfilled lives, rather that they have not been given the linguistic tools they need in order to make sense of their experiences and their conceivings. Not the least of Berger's points is that the way in which society is constructed acts to waste and empty most of the lives it does not destroy.

Berger acknowledges that in order to realize a much more full and equal achievement of human potential it is vital that all people should practise and become proficient in conceiving in the widest possible way so that they will learn to select from a range of theories in response to unique situations and experiences, rather than to act according to set dictates:

> Good general diagnosticians are rare, not because most doctors lack medical knowledge, but because most are incapable of taking in all the possible relevant facts—emotional, historical, environmental as well as physical. They are searching for specific conditions instead of the truth about a man which may then suggest various conditions. It may be that computers will soon diagnose better than doctors. But the facts fed to computers will still have to be the result of intimate, individual recognition of the patient. (Berger and Mohr, 1976, pp. 73–74)

One of the points that Berger is making here is that computers are limited by the theories that they are given to enable them to diagnose. Such theories may be very good diagnostic tools, but they are not the whole story about diagnosis. What is required as well is human involvement and the ability to empathize, to pick up clues and hints, to respond personally, to come to know and understand another human being by being able to imagine oneself in the position of that other person. Berger is talking about the power of conceiving. A power which needs theories but which also goes beyond theory. Of course he knows that the need to develop this power of conceiving is not important only in the case of medical practitioners:

> There are large sections of the English working and middle class who are inarticulate as the result of their wholesale cultural deprivation. They are deprived of the means of translating what they know into thoughts which they can think. They have no examples to follow in which words clarify experience. Their spoken proverbial traditions have long been destroyed: and, although they are literate in the strictly technical sense, they have not had the opportunity of discovering the existence of a written cultural heritage. (Berger and Mohr, 1976, pp. 98–99)

These people can conceive but they cannot translate their ideas into action. Without a 'cultural literacy' there is usually no route from the conceiving to the concept and so to a theory. *Without having had access to an education which goes beyond standard literacy and numeracy, without anything more than a superficial knowledge of theory and language 'ordinary people' are deprived of a full opportunity to assess and to debate inwardly.* They have experience, and practical and intuitive skills, but they do not have the means to develop this knowledge into communicable theories of life.

Berger knows that this argument is not fully testable, but he does not think that this makes his case invalid or wrong:

> What I am saying about Sassall and his patients is subject to the danger which accompanies any imaginative effort. At certain times my own subjectivity may distort. At no time can I prove what I am saying. I can only claim that after years of observation of the subject I believe that what I am saying, despite my clumsiness, reveals a significant part of the social reality of the small area in question, and a large part of the psychological reality of Sassall's life. *The greatest stumbling block to accepting this is the false view that what people cannot express is always simple because they are simple. We like to retain such a view because it confirms our own bogus sense of articulate individuality, and because it saves us from thinking about the extraordinarily complex convergence of philosophical traditions, feelings, half-realised ideas, atavistic instincts, imaginative intimations, which lie behind the simplest hope or disappointment of the simplest person.* (Berger and Mohr, 1976, p. 110) [Italics added]

This argument is the exact opposite of elitism. Berger is describing the unique and remarkable human ability of conceiving. The possession of such an ability indicates the great depth of human beings—even of the ones regarded as 'simple' or 'thick', or any other of the many unkind labels we use. There is great scope for development if only people are given the opportunity—the right circumstances for growth. It is not naive idealism to argue that people should be given the chance to develop themselves to the full—on the contrary, it is the only civilized course to take.

It is worth briefly restating the importance of conceiving. Conceiving creates concepts and theories, and it also depends on them. The more theories a person has, the better equipped he is to conceive. The *power of conceiving* is essential to human individuality, autonomy, and morality. It is not a moral action to follow theory blindly even if it has welcome consequences for other people. Computers cannot be moral even if they are running programs which have moral consequences.

Conceiving draws upon such factors as existing theories, experience, memory, analogy, and imagination. No new theories can be developed wtihout the power of conceiving (try it!). No selection of appropriate aspects of two or more theories is possible without either a further theory or this personal power. In response to unique situations such guiding theories are rare. The unique human ability of conceiving mainly lies fallow within the majority of people, and yet the best practical and moral way of removing obstacles to personal achievement is to encourage self-care and self-development. The general pay-off of this point of view is, initially, at the level of personal maintenance. This is the level at which traditional health education is aimed, where it is hoped that people will become better equipped to take decisions designed to enhance their physical wellbeing. A more far-reaching pay-off of working to develop people's powers of conceiving, theorizing and communicating will be environmental and social change if enough people believe and understand that existing situations and arrangements are acting as impediments to their development.

What benefits could work towards these central aims bring about?

The basic point of health education and promotion is to lay the foundations for self-development in a world of vastly complicated interconnections.

The benefits for 'lay-people'

Given the wider knowledge, competence, and confidence that is necessary for increased self-development there will be:

1. Less feeling of worthlessness.
2. An ability and an inclination to educate other people, to assist others to the stage where they can begin, at whatever level, to develop themselves.
3. The practical opportunities to debate 'health issues'. In other words people will be able to discuss the standards of their own and other people's qualities of life in wide terms.

As far as problems of illness and disease are concerned there will be:

1. Far less need for paternalism by doctors. The reflex response—illness symptoms so, a visit to the doctor so, blind obedience of the doctor's instructions—will be replaced by informed conversation resulting in personal choice.
2. Less dependence on the traditional health services. Those capable of self-care and self-development will demand to look after themselves. As a result there will be less crowded surgery waiting rooms, and reduced hospital waiting-lists.

The benefits for present health care professionals

An appreciation of the arguments put forward here will not only benefit 'lay-people'. The whole range of present health care professionals will gain. Although they will retain their specialist skills *they will also recognize that they have a wider, more generalist role*. The overall emphasis of their work will change—the general focus will be how to encourage and assist people to develop themselves. The most significant of benefits for existing health care professionals will be *intellectual liberation*.

An illustration of this point from the practice of health visiting

Unique situations confront health care professionals constantly. Health visitors have the opportunity to make personal informed judgements frequently, but often are constrained by set rules and procedures. How would a health visitor react to the many problems presented by the James family?

Is the problem medical, environmental, social, psychological, or something else? Where does the health visitor begin to offer solutions? There are no clear rules to follow in such cases as this—different health visitors may well opt for different courses of action. This is a good thing, and not a problem.

Health visiting draws on a range of disciplines because health visitors aim to remove obstacles to people's potentials in their home and family environments. Health visitors learn such theories as those of nutrition, sociology, social policy, psychology, epidemiology, and child development—and in addition they must be qualified nurses—but there is no systematic rationale of health visiting or the teaching of it. Consequently there is a debate in health-visiting circles about the need for a comprehensive theoretical model of health visiting to which all tutors, fieldwork teachers, and practitioners could subscribe. This lack of a coherent model concerns some health visitors who have become accustomed to doing what they have been told to do. It frightens people who are assured by rules.

Mill has made countless telling comments on the topic of rule following. This one is particularly appropriate:

> Thus the mind itself is bowed to the yoke: even in what people do for pleasure, conformity is the first thing thought of; they like in crowds; they exercise choice only among things commonly done: peculiarity of taste, eccentricity of conduct, are shunned equally with crimes: until by dint of not following their own nature they have no nature to follow: their human capacities are withered and starved: they become incapable of any strong wishes or native pleasures, and are generally without either opinions or feelings of home growth, or properly their own. Now is this, or is it not, the desirable condition of human nature? (Mill, 1910, p. 119)

The fear and disorientation experienced by some health visitors is made worse when, as often happens in practice, the various specialist theories are in conflict. Should the James child be given medication and the parents counselled, or should the child be removed from such an environment? Should they be rehoused, or should they be shown how to get things changed on their own behalf? Should Mr James be made to do community work instead of his probation, or should something be done about getting him a proper job? How is the health visitor to choose the most appropriate course of action in such a complex case in the absence of a guiding theory? The Council for the Education and Training of Health Visitors puts the problem in this way:

> Much literature relevant to health visiting is descriptive; very little explains how to do health visiting. Principles are implied but rarely examined or made explicit. For this reason theories and methods taught can only be . . . (those) . . . of individual tutors based on their own personal experience. Lack of security in health visiting theory is a problem for fieldwork teachers who have the explicit responsibility of correlating theory with practice. How can I correlate theory with practice for a student when neither of us seems to know what the theory is? (CETHV, 1977)

It is at such points that the power of conceiving—which will often be called 'commonsense'—is invoked to synthesize such elements as theories, empathies, past experience, discussions with colleagues, and common humanity. What is missing is not competence but individual confidence to shake off a debilitating reverence for specific theories and rules. As things stand health visitors are often confused, uncertain, and lack confidence. They feel that they are doing wrong by not following set prescriptions for action and as a result can, because they feel they have to, invoke preferred specific theories which seem the least irrelevant in given situations, but which, because they are specific, may not produce the best results. Many health visitors do not have the confidence to take an overall view of their practice. They look at a situation and are taught to make lists of single aims and objectives, when they really need a wider more flexible and fluid approach, constantly bearing in mind their fundamental *enabling* role. The central question for health visitors should always be 'how can I enable this individual or family best, how can I get them to the point where they can work to develop themselves?' Certainly specific obstacles will need to be eliminated—such as the bronchitis and the damp—but these obstacles should not be thought of in isolation from the wider problem. Health is equivalent to the set of conditions which fulfil, or enable an individual to work to fulfil, his biological and chosen potentials. The issue of how to create better health is never clear-cut— this basic point should never be forgotten. By splitting the task of health creation into specific domains and objectives there is a real danger that the wider aim will be neglected. Theories must be used, but they should not be used apart from the power of conceiving.

Dingwall (1977) has argued:

> Doctors don't worry about a theory of medicine; engineers don't worry about a theory of engineering. They follow courses which the practitioner may then use in a personal synthesis to meet the demands of any individual situation. (Dingwall, 1977)

The other benefits for present health care professionals, whatever their specialism, are that they will recognize the need to add to the width of their conceiving. Since their careers are dedicated to the removal of obstacles to the achievement of human potential they should work to understand more theories, and to gain more experience relevant to their wide vocations. Unless good reasons are advanced to show this to be counter productive this recognition will lead to a breakdown, or at least a blurring of, the demarcations between specialisms.

The final benefit will be of their fundamental role as educators. Ignorance is wasting and the catalyst of fear. In all cases of contact with clients; theories, alternatives, consequences and choices should be explained. This may be time consuming in the short-term, but if practised always and universally will have significant long-term benefits.

Summary and Conclusions

The aim of health education and promotion is, in general, to bring the individual — and so to bring groups of individuals — to the level where they have the best sets of background conditions for his, her or their chosen and biological potentials. Health education and promotion is about creating *choices*. Health education should go further than is traditional, both in the training of the professionals and in the education which they try to provide in turn. Full health education is not just to do with creating traditional health choices about such things as smoking and exercise, and it is not only to do with creating choices at the level of a one-to-one relationship with a client. Education for and the promotion of health goes far wider than this.

1. At the individual level health education is to do with making people as fully aware as possible about the factors which can affect their basic foundations for achievement. Because of this, full health education must ensure that people understand about the causes of disease and illness, but also that they are politically literate — that they have a knowledge of the institutions and policies which shape their lives. If people have poor levels of general education then health education should work to remedy this.

Also it should do more than this. It should teach people to face questions directly, and to think for themselves. *It should aim to develop people's powers of conceiving.* Education for health is work for wholeness. It is not just to do with physical functioning, it is at least equally to do with the mental life of a person. It is misleading to speak of 'health potential' or 'health status' with their present limited meaning. This usage tends to focus attention solely on biological potential, but work for health in its full and proper sense is work towards laying the foundations for full human flourishing. This is what a true health service should be aiming to do. The removal of the obstacles of illness and disease is only one aspect of true work for health. True health education should work to enable people to understand better what they are, what they believe, and what they know. It should seek people's opinions and it should enable discussion. The last thing that health education should do is to treat people like babies. People are tremendously complicated and often devastatingly underdeveloped. People need to be challenged. We need to be forced to face our worlds.

As Mill has written:

> The human faculties of perception; judgement, discriminative feeling, mental activity, and even moral preference, are exercised only in making a choice. He who does anything because it is custom makes no choice. He gains no practice either in discerning or in desiring what is best. The mental and moral, like the muscular powers, are improved only by being used. (Mill, 1910, pp. 116–117)

2. Just as full health education has to involve political education and not indoctrination, health promotion has to involve political action. 'Health for All' will

not have been achieved even in a situation where all members of a society have optimum physical fitness if other foundations for the achievement of potential are weak, and other human potentials restricted.

The acknowledgement that political literacy and action are a part of work for health should not be thought to be the pollution of an otherwise pure discipline. Traditional health care is not removed from politics. For example, political ideals underlie the present tensions between the National Health Service and the private provision of 'health care'. Decisions about the funding of the National Health Service are taken by politicians. Political decisions are taken about the roles of medicine and health education. Not to provide a more positive and comprehensive service is both overtly and tacitly a political act. To maintain the present system in the face of alternatives is a political decision.

There are so many factors which influence people's basic foundations for achievement. Such factors as racial discrimination, grossly unequal distribution of income and power, inadequate housing, a poor education service, and low levels of fulfilling employment all have a significant bearing on the quality of people's lives. Promotion and education for health consequently involves explaining and publicizing these influences, highlighting particular problems, suggesting alternatives, pressing for change, writing articles, writing letters to the press, and pushing these ideas amongst other professionals. The publications *Radical Health Promotion* and *Radical Health Visitor*, produced on shoestring budgets, are examples of these very things.

This task should not fall only on those of one political belief. There is room for many different ideals in health creation. It may be that people who incline towards the beliefs of the Tory Party, and groups even further to the right, will be less keen and less able to do these things. But, if they are truly to work for health, if they are to create equitable foundations for achievement, then this is what they must do. To argue that eventually the best foundations will be laid by getting rid of all foundations—by doing such things as dismantling the welfare state, by providing only basic vocational training, by cutting state benefits, and by cutting the funding of present enabling services—so that the strongest will flourish, create wealth, and then hand some of it back to those who do not have foundations, is immoral, selfish, nonsense. It is immoral because there can be no morality without choice, and to remove all foundations is effectively to remove all meaningful choice from many people. It is selfish because it permits unfettered self-interest *at the expense of others*. And it is nonsense because the habitually self-motivated cannot, and do not wish to, make a sudden conversion to the sacrifices—in money, in time, and in thinking about other people as one would think about oneself—involved in caring for and providing the basic needs of others.

Chapter Nine
How Can Health
for All be Achieved?

This should not be the final chapter but the first. The question requires, and has received throughout history, considerable thought and argument. In one sense the answer to the question is simple. How can health for all be achieved? Answer: Such a state can never be achieved. Health for all cannot be achieved because Utopias cannot be achieved. People inevitably suffer, are sick, and have other problems. Different people have different values and priorities: the world is such that there will always be winners and losers. In another sense the answer to the question is vastly complicated.

How can health for all be achieved? Answers: By revolutions—bloody, intellectual, or some other kind. By democratic processes—by slow change from within. By direct political action to redistribute wealth and power. By extending true education. By civil warfare—as in South Africa, a country which collectively has an appallingly low standard of health. By changing the various fixed institutions of societies. By legal reforms. By economic change. By group pressure. By working to extend the range of ideas of individuals. By some combination of all or some of these answers. It makes sense to propose these sorts of answers if health is seen in the light of the theory which has been put forward in this book. If a person's health is equivalent to the state of his set of foundations for achievement, then the issue is not—how can a Utopia be created?—but how can *equitable minimum conditions to enable people to achieve fulfilling lives* be created? How can the *central conditions* which make up health be best provided for all people?

The discussion about how health for all is to be created is not fundamentally to do with questions about the meanings of words, even though these questions should never be allowed to slip into the background. The discussion must take place at the level of political and social theory and policy. It cannot be denied that people possess a great range of potentials, the question is *what system will bring the most of them to fruition?* This question spawns a million others: where will the money come from? Who is to suffer and who is to impose the sacrifices which will be required of some people? What degree of coercion is permissible in order to bring about the ultimately liberating changes? Can defence and medical spending be cut to provide an improved education service? Should single societies aim to create the minimum conditions, and then work to help other societies, or should work for health be constantly global?

There is a seemingly infinite minefield of theoretical and policy dilemmas to negotiate. These have to be considered and explained, and decisions have to be reached, but it should never be forgotten that now, in the real world, people are shamefully ignorant, underdeveloped, badly fed, badly housed, and saturated with indoctrination.

Debate and discussion should not conceal the need for action now, at whatever level, aimed to improve the health of all people, whether they are friends, neighbours, strangers, or enemies. There is always something, however small, that can be done to enable someone to achieve more than otherwise would have been the case. This is what matters most. We need to think, to work out ways of providing more of this service.

CONCLUSION

Although the major theme of this inquiry has been to understand more about the complexity of the meaning of health, and of the various implications of the theories of health, it has also tried to lay a foundation of its own. Unless it is seriously mistaken, the new theory of health demonstrates that work for health is often controversial and never a question of following ordained guidelines unthinkingly. *Work for health inevitably requires thought and reflection about which course of action is the most appropriate to a particular situation in which assistance of some sort is to be given.* Work for health in itself should create more health in the workers.

This book has tried to bury the myth that the goal of 'health for all' is solely or primarily the concern of medical science. Medicine should be seen as one way, amongst many others, of working to create health. It is not necessarily the most important.

This is a major consequence of the theory advanced in this book. The general argument only scratches the surface of an intensely complex, perhaps not fully penetrable, problem about how to improve the general quality of human existence. But, as far as ideas about the nature of health are concerned, at least it scratches deeper than has been scratched before. There are so many controversies which arise out of the book, so many unanswered questions, and so much has not been properly thought through, that it is truly inadequate. But in some places it is stronger than others and it is here that any critics should concentrate. If health is not to do with the quality of human life then what is it to do with? If health is properly and exclusively the concern of medicine and paramedicine, why is this so?

Appendix
Objectivity

This appendix has been included because issues of objectivity appear in various places in the book. It is not a central issue, but it is hardly ever out of the picture. It is now often taken for granted that strong objectivity is not possible, and that 'values permeate everything', but why this is so is not often considered or explained. It is important in the context of this book to show that it is mistaken to believe that one human being—for instance, a doctor, a health educator, or a nurse—can ever be fully detached from another human being—for instance, a patient or a client. Many practitioners rightly regard their work as a craft—a personal skill which uses some of the tools of science, but which also goes beyond science.

The view that any inquiry, even 'scientific inquiry', can be detached, impartial, and objective is incorrect. In all inquiry the unquantifiable, human, creative, emotional, intuitive, caring, egoistic, competitive element is indispensable. If this is so with chemicals then it must be many times more so with people, who are more than the sum of chemical components. The idea of 'total objectivity' is a myth which can be shown to be so once and for all, with a consequent emphasis on our shared humanity.

This view of objectivity does not entail that any theory is as good as any other. There are always some standards to be met. If it is not possible to claim that a theory is 'objective' and therefore must be correct, then other questions have to be asked. For example one might ask, is this theory preferred because it is more practical, more simple, more consistent, more effective, more fruitful, cheaper to apply, or easier to explain? Does it accord with prevailing views in its own and other disciplines? Whichever questions seem most appropriate must be asked. For instance, in the case of health it is necessary to ask whether a particular theory acts to remove obstacles in a way that is better than any alternative theory, rather than to ask whether this theory is 'objectively correct'.

The traditional view of objectivity is that it involves a 'detached attitude'. This view is thought to draw on the best features of genuine inquiry. On this view 'objective inquiries' are impartial and concerned with the 'raw truth'. Another sense must be added if this theory is to be at all realistic, but in so doing the overall view is shown to be inconsistent. The sense to be added is that of consensus belief. According to this sense objectivity can be said to have been achieved when there is agreed belief amongst all, or almost all, informed people.

There are therefore three senses of objectivity according to this new view (see the accompanying diagram). As these senses and the connections between them are explained the example of journalistic inquiry is used in the main. The same general points apply to all inquiry including scientific inquiry but journalism provides a more accessible and topical means of illustration. *Sense A* is the idea of an 'objective attitude', of neutrality towards the evidence. Journalists and scientists sometimes claim this

OBJECTIVITY

Is DETACHMENT the general sense?

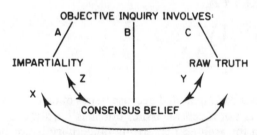

Sense *A* is the idea of an 'objective attitude', of *neutrality* towards evidence.

Sense *B* is the idea that objectivity is assured by expert agreement;

Sense *C* is the notion of an 'absolute truth', a truth *apart* from human beings. Events, circumstances and facts as they would be without human interpretation.

But: X — How can 'raw truth' be discovered without conceiving, theories, choosing, deciding, and selecting evidence?

Y — What guarantee is there that 'raw truth' has been discovered even if all experts agree?

Z — Beliefs (which are necessary for any understanding) are, by definition, partial (a choice will have been made to prefer one belief, or set of beliefs, over other possible beliefs). It is not possible to hold a belief impartially.

(With apologies to Stuart Brown, author of Unit 14, Open University course U202 and reproduced by permission of the Open University.)

neutrality, arguing that they are impartial or indifferent to the evidence which they record. *Sense B* is the idea that objectivity is assured by expert agreement. *Sense C* is the notion of an 'absolute truth', a truth apart from human beings: events, circumstances, and facts as they would be without human interpretation.

There are problems associated with inquiring and reporting 'objectively' according to the spirit of each single sense. The coupling of these senses by the double arrows serves to highlight these difficulties. To take the double arrow marked X first of all. The implication for journalists of this coupling is: *When a journalist inquires objectively he reports impartially and so uncovers the truth.* But journalists are bound to select. It can be agreed that journalists will uncover evidence and they will be able to write reports about which other journalists will agree, but they will not uncover the 'raw truth', nor will they have investigated impartially. Just as it can be said that art comes into being through interpretation (as Gadamer thinks) so it can be said that 'facts' come into being only when evidence and interpretation combine.

The 'raw truth' must be every factor of whatever type that has a bearing on the report that is written. If the report is of a battle in a war it is clearly not possible to select every aspect which has some relationship to that battle, similarly with a report of an industrial dispute, and similarly with a report about a wedding written for the local rag. To report the 'raw truth' would take forever. All journalists will have been briefed and/or will have undertaken some research prior to the investigation. This being so they will have arrived at whatever event on which they are to report armed with certain theories, say, about which aspects are the most important, the most effective and pertinent questions to ask, and about who is the best person to answer these questions. Journalists are *bound* to be selective about the evidence they amass, and about their treatment of it, even about weddings, and the same point holds for all inquiry however serious its nature. Certain photographs and film sequences will be felt to be more significant than others, certain phrases will be felt to be more full of meaning; and these things will inevitably be selected according, at least in part, to prior beliefs about significance and meaningfulness in that particular type of situation. Quite simply, decisions must be made about what is relevant and these decisions cannot be made according to the dictates of the theory of strong objectivity, which holds that decisions can be made impartially.

The art of succinct summary, précis and editing is crucial to good journalism— and good science—and it is the nature of making a précis when there are no specifiable rules to govern that précis, that it can be done only by people who have a view about what they are shortening; it can be done only by people who understand the meaning of the piece. If journalists are truly impartial then they will not be able to decide where to begin their inquiries since all evidence will have to be afforded equal merit. Journalists could be replaced by non-discriminating machines such as videos and tape-recorders (although even these machines are limited in certain ways and cannot therefore record the 'whole truth'). Darwin recognized the problem. Writing in the 1860s he said, 'About thirty years ago there was much talk that geologists ought only to observe and not to theorize; and I can well remember saying that at this rate a man might as well go into a gravel pit and count the pebbles and describe the colours.'

Are the following 'objective statements' according to the theory of strong objectivity? 'The cause of cancer is directly related to the presence of an angiogenic factor in particular areas of the body': 'Mountain ranges are the effect of Continental Drift': 'Arthur Scargill spoke out strongly in defence of the NUM's hard-line': 'Schizophrenia is a mental illness marked by disconnected thoughts, feelings, and actions. It is associated with delusions and a retreat from social life'? They are not. A selection has been made from a body of evidence.

The problem associated with double arrow Y is the general problem that the consensus of human opinion about the true nature of physical reality is in itself no guarantee of knowledge of the actual true nature. This point has been noticed by many historians and philosophers of science who have charted the continual change in human theories about reality. The most well-known example of all is that it was once universally believed that the Sun orbited the Earth rather than vice versa: agreement is no guarantee of truth.

Double arrow Z completes the picture. If groups of journalists are agreed in their beliefs, or even if one single journalist has a belief, then that group of journalists, or that journalist, is necessarily partial. A decision has been made to prefer one possible belief over other possibilities. Consequently there is an incompatibility between the sense of objectivity being that of impartiality, and the sense of objectivity as being consensus belief. The fundamental point here is that it is impossible to have an impartial belief: if something is believed then it is believed in preference to alternatives.

What this analysis emphasizes is the role of human beings in deciding what is thought to be 'objective'. It emphasizes shared humanity and individual responsibility for decisions. It is an error to argue that there is ever only one 'right decision' to be made in medicine or health care. This is a salutory realization for people who believe that what they see (or perceive as a problem) compels their actions. This can be the case but it can also be that how a person thinks affects that person's perceptions and actions. All inquiry is done by partial human beings; descriptions and explanations depend not only on raw evidence but also on human beliefs about that evidence. Factors peculiar to human beings affect reporting, theorizing, conceiving, and in a medical context, the selection of drugs for prescription, diagnosis, clinical practice and curriculum design, for instance. These practices cannot ultimately be based on purely objective grounds.

References and Further Reading

Bacon, F. (1905) *The Philosophical Works*. Robertson (ed.). Routledge, London.

Berger, J., and Mohr, J. (1976) *A Fortunate Man*. Writers & Readers Publishing Cooperative, London.

Black (1982) *Inequalities in Health: the Black Report*. Penguin, Harmondsworth.

Brody, H. (1973) 'The Systems View of Man: Implications for Medicine, Science, and Ethics.' In *Perspectives in Biology and Medicine,*

An all-encompassing view of man seen as 'a hierarchy of . . . natural systems interconnected by various patterns of information flow in feedback circuits'. This idea aims to incorporate every aspect of man from atoms (micro) to the biosphere (macro). Consequently, ' "Health" may then be defined as the harmonious interaction of all hierarchical components while "disease" is the result of a force which perturbs or disrupts hierarchical structure.'

Such extreme utopianism distracts from the substantial point that all aspects of existence, not only the personal, can have a bearing on the quality of individual life.

Caplan, A. L., Englehardt, H. T., Jr., and McCartney, J. J. (eds.) (1981) *Concepts of Health and Disease: Interdisciplinary Perspectives*. Addison-Wesley Publishing Company, Reading, MA.

This book is a comprehensive 'reader' which does much to fill in further details of 'the approach of medical science' and 'the sociological approach'. Several of the papers attempt to distinguish between 'health' and 'disease', and agree that such questions are never value-free. However, since it is such a large collection of contributions there are many unresolved conflicts between the various authors, and several keywords are used ambiguously.

Council for the Education and Training of Health Visitors (1977) *An Investigation into the Principle of Health Visiting*.

Cribb, A. (1986) *Politics and Health in the School Curriculum*. In Watt, A. and Rodmell, S. Routledge and Kegan Paul, London.

Culver, C. M., and Gert, B. (1982) *Philosophy in Medicine*. Oxford University Press, New York.

A fine introduction to philosophical analysis. The book aims to clarify a number of central questions in medicine, including the nature of 'disease' and 'illness', the nature of 'consent' and 'competence', possible justifications of 'paternalism', and the definition and criterion of 'death'.

De Jong, G. A., and Rutten, F. F. H. (1983) 'Justice and Health for All'. *Social Science and Medicine*, **17**(14) 1085–1095.

A clear explanation of a typical sociological view of health.

Dingwall, R. (1977) *The Social Organisation of Health Visitor Training*. Croom Helm, London.

Doyal, L., and Pennell, I. (1979). *The Political Economy of Health*. Pluto Press, London.

This readable book questions the view that illness and disease are misfortunes that just happen to people, and which scientific medicine is dedicated to combating. The main argument is that 'ill-health' in both developed and under-developed countries is largely a product of the social and economic organization of society.

Dubos, R. (1959) *The Mirage of Health*. Harper and Row, New York.

Feyerabend, P. (1978) *Against Method*. Verso, London. Recommended reading for all those addicted to rule following.

Field, D. (1976) 'The Social Definition of Illness'. In Tuckett, D. (1976).

Foucault, M. (1973) *The Birth of the Clinic*. (Translated from the French by A. M. Sheridan Smith.) Tavistock, London.

Gallie, W. B. (1964) *Philosophy and the Historical Understanding*. Chatto and Windus, London.

Gorz, A. (1983) *Ecology as Politics*. Pluto Press, London.

Greaves, D. (1979). 'What is Medicine? Towards a Philosophical Approach', *Journal of Medical Ethics*, **5**, pp. 29–32.

> This is an important paper written by a practising physician. Greaves's argument is that there is a crisis in medicine which either requires or will initiate a 'paradigm change'. He lists seven points which he thinks are indicative of a crisis. These include the fact that chronic intractable conditions exist which medicine can only marginally affect, definition of legitimate areas of concern for health professionals is problematic, the need to re-emphasize a personal rather than a technical approach, an increasing desire of people to be informed and to take part in decision making, and diminishing confidence in technological solutions. Greaves concludes that a conscious effort must be made to change the existing situation. He argues that medicine must be envisaged as free from the notion of diseases as things, and that the implications of a return to the alternative approach, which makes the sick individual the focus so that his illness is inseparable from him and his diseases alone are no longer recognizable, must be explored. Such a task would require the involvement of all those disciplines which are currently challenging medicine, together with a new commitment to an interdisciplinary approach.

Illich, I. (1977) *Limits to Medicine*. Pelican Books, London

Kennedy, I. (1981) *The Unmasking of Medicine*. George Allen & Unwin, London.

King, L. S. (1954) 'What is Disease?' *Philosophy of Science*, **21**, 193–203.

Koestler, A. (1969) *The Act of Creation*. Hutchinson, London.

Lloyd Jones, E. (1891) 'Further Observations on the Specific Gravity of the Blood in Health and Disease', *Journal of Physiology*, **12**, 299–346.

Mansfield, K. (1977) *Letters and Journals*, Pelican Books, London.

Meador, C. (1965) 'The Art and Science of Non-disease', *New England Journal of Medicine*, **272**, 92–95

Mechanic, D. (1962) 'The Concept of Illness Behaviour', *Journal of Chronic Diseases*, **15**, 189–194.

Mill, J. S. (1910) *Utilitarianism, On Liberty, and Considerations on Representative Government*. Dent, London.

Mitchell, J. (1984) *What is to be done about Illness and Health?* Penguin, Harmondsworth.

O'Neill, P. (1983) *Health Crisis 2000*. Heinemann, London.

Open Univeristy (1981) Second Level Course, *Inquiry*, U202, Open University Press, Milton Keynes

Open University (1985) Second Level Course, *Issues in Health and Disease*, U205, Open University Press, Milton Keynes.

> Useful on statistical analysis, biology and epidemiology. Concerned with study of disease not health.

Parsons, T. (1981) 'Definitions of Health and Illness in the Light of American Values and Social Structure'. In Caplan *et al.* (1981).

Partridge, E. (1966) *Origins*. Routledge & Kegan Paul, London.

Peery, T. M., and Miller, F. N. (1971) *Pathology*, 2nd ed. Little, Brown, Boston.

Plato. *The Republic*.

Plato. *The Last Days of Socrates*.

Polanyi, M. (1973). *Personal Knowledge*. Routledge & Kegan Paul, London.

Popper, K. (1973) *Objective Knowledge*. Oxford University Press, Oxford.

Sacks, O. (1982) *Awakenings*. Picador, Pan Books, London.

Seedhouse, D. F. (1984) *Rationality*. PhD thesis. Manchester University.

Sigerist, H. E. (1970) *Civilisation and Disease*. University of Chicago Press, Chicago.

Solzhenitsyn, A. (1971) *Cancer Ward*. Penguin, London.

Stacey, M. (1976) *Concepts of Health and Illness: A working paper*. The University of Warwick.

Stacey, M. (1980) *Sociological Concepts of Health and Disease and Critiques of Such Concepts*.
    Both are reviews of the literature in medical sociology which deals with 'concepts of
    health and illness'. Discussion of the differences between individualistic and collectivist
    'models of health'. Useful introductions to the sociological debate.

Tuckett, D. (ed.) (1976) *An Introduction to Medical Sociology*. Tavistock, London.

Waitzin, H. (1978) 'A Marxist View of Medical Care', *Annals of Internal Medicine*, **89**,
    264–278.
    A Marxist perspective. This Marxist view questions whether major improvements in
    the health care system can occur without fundamental changes in broad social order.

White, W. A. (1926) *The Meaning of Disease*. Williams and Wilkins, Baltimore.

Williams, R. (1976) *Keywords*. Fontana/Croom Helm, London.

Williams, R. (1983) 'Concepts of health: An analysis of lay logic'. *Sociology*, **17**(2), 185–205.

Wilson, M. (1975) *Health is for People*. Darton, Longman and Todd.

Wittgenstein, L. (1974) *Philosophical Investigations*. Basil Blackwell, Oxford.

World Health Organization. (1946) *Constitution*. WHO, Geneva.

Zola, I. K. (1972) 'Medicine as an institution of social control, *Sociological Review*, **20**(4),
    487–509.

Index